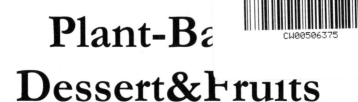

Plant-Based Dessert&Fruits

Cook Fantastic Plant-Based Dessert!

Carolyn J. Perez

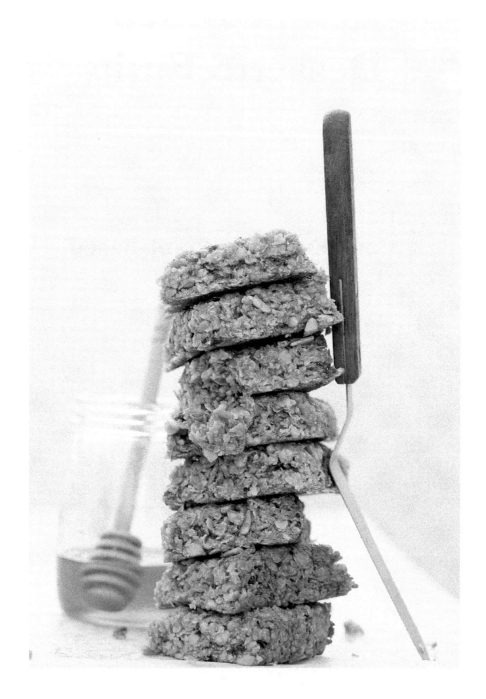

This Book Included

Book 1:

PLANT-BASED DESSERT&FRUITS

Easy, healthy, tasty Plant-Based dessert recipes to stay fit with taste!

Book 2:

PLANT-BASED DESSERT

Super tasty vegetable and fruit based dessert recipes to lose weight with taste!

Carolyn J. Perez

Plant-Based

Dessert & Fruits

Easy, healthy, tasty Plant-Based Dessert recipes to stay fit with taste!

Carolyn J. Perez

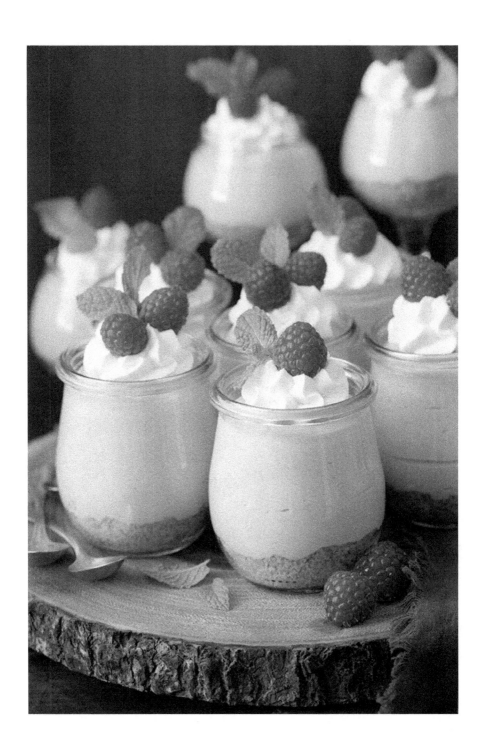

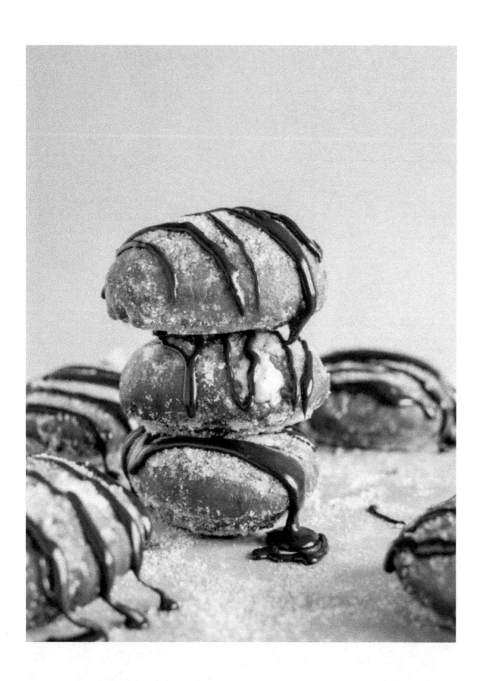

Contents

Introduction

It is a common thought to think that following a diet is necessarily linked to the concept of actual weight loss. However, this is not always the case: following a diet is often directly linked to the foods that we decide to include in our tables daily.

In addition, we do not always choose the best quality ingredients to cook our dishes.

Sometimes we are so rushed and unruly that we forget that we love our bodies. And what better cure than a healthy diet? Following a healthy diet should become more than an imposition or a punishment, but a real lifestyle.

Moreover, this is the Plant-based diet goal: not to impose a restrictive and sometimes impossible diet to follow, but to recreate a diet based on foods of natural origin and above all healthy. Therefore, the plant based represents a real food trend. However, as we will see it is much more than just a fashion trend, but a real lifestyle.

In addition, it is the aim of this text, or rather of this cookbook, to introduce you to the plant based discipline. And we will do it with a few theoretical explanations, just to make you understand what we are talking about and above all how to prepare it: there will be a purely practical part where you will find 50 recipes on the plant based. These recipes will be divided into appetizers, snacks, first and second courses, side dishes and finally a string of plant based desserts.

In the end, you will be spoiled for choice to start following this healthy dietary discipline.

Plant based diet: what are we talking about?

We already mentioned that more than a real weight loss diet the Plant based diet is a food discipline. Food discipline is enjoying great success not only because it is very fashionable, but because it applies such principles that can be perfectly integrated into our daily lives. The plant-based diet is a true approach to life, starting with nutrition: respect for one's health and body, first of all, which is reflected in respect for all forms of life and the planet in general.

As the word itself says, it deals with a food plan based, precisely on what comes from plants. However, simply calling it that way would be too simplistic.

It is a predominantly plant-based diet, but not only. It is not just about consuming vegetables but about taking natural foods: not industrially processed, not treated, and not deriving from the exploitation of resources and animals, preferably zero km.

So it could be a discipline that aims not only at environmental saving but also at the economic one: think about what advantages, in fact, at the level of your pockets you can have if you apply the principle of 0Km and therefore to be able to harvest your vegetables directly from your garden.

Environmental savings do not only mean pollution reduction: the ethical component (present exclusively in the vegan diet, for example) is combined with a strong will to health. This means that the plant based, in addition to not preferring foods that exploit animals, is also based on foods that are especially unprocessed, fresh, healthy, balanced, light, and rich in essential nutrients. In practice, it is a plant-based diet but not vegan / vegetarian, emphasizing the quality and wholesomeness of foods rather than on their moral value, albeit with great attention to sustainability. Such a lifestyle could therefore be of help, not only to our health, but also to create a more sustainable world for future generations.

Main differences between Vegan and Plant based diet

The plant-based diet is often associated with the vegan diet.
This is because both plan to include cruelty free foods that
do not involve any animal exploitation.

Furthermore, they are associated precisely because they are
both predominantly plant-based.

However, there are some pretty obvious differences between
these two diets.

First of all, precisely for the reasoning behind the prevalence
of plants.

It is well known that even the vegan diet provides a diet
based on foods of plant origin: unlike the plant-based diet,
however, nothing of animal derivation is allowed, neither
direct nor indirect, nor other products - clothing or
accessories - which include the exploitation of animals.

No eggs, no milk, no honey, no leather, so to speak, and not
only: in its most rigorous meanings, veganism does not even
include the use of yeasts, as the bacteria that compose them
are indisputably living beings.

A vegan diet can be balanced if the person who leads it knows well the foods and their combinations, the necessary supplements, and their body's reaction to the lack of certain foods.

On the contrary, the Plant-Based diet is on the one hand more relaxed, on the other more stringent.

What does it mean?

This means that it is on the one hand more relaxed because it is plant-based, but not exclusively vegetable: products of animal origin are allowed, in moderate quantities, but under only one condition, namely the excellent quality of the food itself and its certified origin. For example, eggs can be consumed occasionally but only if very fresh, possibly at zero km, from free-range farms where the hens are not exploited but can live outdoors without constraints.

It is also a somewhat more stringent philosophy than veganism precisely for this reason: as long as it is 100% vegetable, the vegan also consumes heavily processed foods, such as industrial fries. Therefore, the vegan can also eat junk foods or snacks. Conversely, plant-based dieters would never admit highly refined foods of this type.

Both dietary approaches are conscious and do not involve the consumption of meat. However, if vegans are driven by ethical reasons, those who follow a plant-based diet also reject everything processed on an industrial level and unhealthy.

A plant-based diet is a diet that aims to eliminate industrially processed foods and, therefore, potentially more harmful to health. It is based on the consumption of fruit and vegetables, whole grains and avoiding (or minimizing) animal products and processed foods. This means that vegan desserts made with refined sugar or bleached flour are also covered.

There is also a substantial difference between the philosophies behind the two diets. As we said in the previous paragraph and above, the ethical component, which is based on the refusal of any food of animal origin, plays a lot in veganism. While for the plant based is not a purely moral and moralistic discourse but on the real thought of being able to keep healthy with the food discipline and be respectful of the environment surrounding us.

Plant based diet full shopping list. What to eat and what to avoid

Now we can examine the complete shopping list of the plant based diet.

Let's briefly summarize the principles on which this particular type of diet is based:

- Emphasizes whole, minimally processed foods.
- Limits or avoids animal products.
- Focuses on plants, including vegetables, fruits, whole grains, legumes, seeds and nuts, which should make up most of what you eat.
- Excludes refined foods, like added sugars, white flour and processed oils.
- Pays special attention to food quality, promoting locally sourced, organic food whenever possible.

As for what you can usually eat, we can say the general consumption of:

- Wholegrain and flours
- extra virgin olive oil

- Seasonal fruit and vegetables: these foods are the basis of every meal.

- In this diet you can also eat sweets but only and exclusively homemade and with controlled raw materials, simple and not very refined, preferably of vegetable origin - for example by replacing milk with soy or rice drinks, and eggs with other natural thickeners such as flaxseed, or simple ripe banana.

- You can also consume nuts and seeds.

As for absolutely forbidden foods, there are all those ready-made and processed:

- ready-made sauces
- chips
- biscuits
- various kinds of snacks
- sugary cereals,
- Spreads, snacks and many other notoriously unhealthy foods.
- Junk food and fast food are therefore absolutely banned
- Sugar beverages

Regarding the complete shopping list:

- Fruits: Berries, citrus fruits, pears, peaches, pineapple, bananas, etc.

- Vegetables: Kale, spinach, tomatoes, broccoli, cauliflower, carrots, asparagus, peppers, etc.

- Starchy vegetables: Potatoes, sweet potatoes, butternut squash, etc.

- Whole grains: Brown rice, rolled oats, spelt, quinoa, brown rice pasta, barley, etc.

- Healthy fats with omega 3: Avocados, olive oil, coconut oil, unsweetened coconut, etc.

- Legumes: Peas, chickpeas, lentils, peanuts, beans, black beans, etc.

- Seeds, nuts and nut butter: Almonds, cashews, macadamia nuts, pumpkin seeds, sunflower seeds, natural peanut butter, tahini, etc.

- Unsweetened plant-based milk: Coconut milk, almond milk, cashew milk, etc.

- Spices, herbs and seasonings: Basil, rosemary, turmeric, curry, black pepper, salt, etc.

- Condiments: Salsa, mustard, nutritional yeast, soy sauce, vinegar, lemon juice, etc.

- Plant-based protein: Tofu, tempeh, seitan, and plant based protein sources or powders with no added sugar or artificial ingredients.
- Beverages: Coffee, tea, sparkling water, etc.

There is the chance to add food of animal origin very rarely, for example if you have specific nutritional needs or if it has been strongly recommended by your doctor. Anyway, if supplementing your plant-based diet with animal products choose quality products from grocery stores or, better yet, purchase them from local farms.

- Eggs: Pasture-raised when possible.
- Poultry: Free-range, organic when possible.
- Beef and pork: Pastured or grass-fed when possible.
- Seafood: Wild-caught from sustainable fisheries when possible.
- Dairy: Organic dairy products from pasture-raised animals whenever possible.

Dessert and fruit recipes

Pumpkin coconut and chocolate cake

PREPARATION TIME: 15 minutes
COOKING TIME: 65 minutes
CALORIES: 455

INGREDIENTS FOR 8 SERVINGS

- 250 grams of already cleaned pumpkin

- 240 grams of wholemeal flour

- 160 grams of raw cane vegan sugar

- 100 g of sunflower oil

- 80 grams of coconut milk

- 1 sachet of yeast (based on cream of tartar)

- ½ teaspoon of cinnamon

- ½ teaspoon of powdered ginger

- 1 pinch of pepper

- 1 pinch of salt

- 30 grams of chopped vegan chocolate

- Coconut flour (to decorate)

DIRECTIONS

1. Clean the pumpkin by removing all the seeds and internal filaments with a spoon.

2. With a sharp knife cut the pumpkin into 2-3 cm thick slices and remove the peel.

3. Weigh 250 grams of cleaned pumpkin and arrange the slices on a baking sheet lined with parchment paper.

4. Bake in a static oven at 180 ° C for 25 minutes, then remove from the oven and let it cool.

5. Now you can move on to preparing the dough.

6. In the food processor, blend the roasted pumpkin until smooth.

7. Pour the wholemeal flour, vegan brown sugar, yeast, cinnamon, ginger, pepper and salt into a bowl.

8. Stir with a wooden spoon then add the pumpkin puree, sunflower oil and coconut milk and mix well.

9. Peel and chop the vegan chocolate.

10. Pour the mixture into a 22 cm diameter cake pan lined with parchment paper.

11. Sprinkle the surface with the chopped almonds and bake in a static oven at 190° C for 40 minutes.

12. Remove from the oven and let cool completely before serving.

13. Serve with a sprinkle of coconut flour.

Banana pear and spelt flour cake

PREPARATION TIME: 15 minutes
COOKING TIME: 65 minutes
CALORIES: 430

INGREDIENTS FOR 6/8 SERVINGS

- 400 grams of wholemeal spelt flour

- 150 grams of vegan brown sugar

- 270 ml of spelt milk

- 1 teaspoon of apple cider vinegar

- 120 grams of sunflower oil

- 1 sachet of natural leavening powder

- 2 ripe bananas

- 2 pears

DIRECTIONS

1. First, put the dose of vinegar in the spelt milk: this will allow the vegetable drink to curdle and thicken, making the dough much softer.

2. In a large bowl, sift the wholemeal spelt flour and baking powder.

3. Then add the brown sugar and mix all the dry ingredients together.

4. Peel bananas and make the pulp.

5. Wash and peel pears too.

6. Proceed by mashing the pulp of the bananas with a fork and cut the pear into cubes.

7. Add the liquid ingredients to the powders, i.e. the curdled spelt milk and sunflower oil, and mix well until you get a smooth consistency.

8. Add the banana pulp and the cut pears, continuing to mix until the fruit is incorporated into the mixture.

9. Pour everything into a baking pan that you have previously oiled and floured.

10. Bake in a static oven at 190 ºC for about 30 minutes.

11. Always check the cooking, and as soon as it is cooked, let it cool.

12. Slice and serve.

Banana and cocoa cake

PREPARATION TIME: 15 minutes
COOKING TIME: 65 minutes
CALORIES: 430

INGREDIENTS FOR 6/8 SERVINGS

- 350 grams of wholemeal flour
- 50 grams of cocoa powder
- 150 grams of vegan brown sugar
- 270 ml of almond milk
- 120 grams of sunflower oil
- 1 sachet of natural leavening powder
- 3 ripe bananas

DIRECTIONS

1. First, in a large bowl, sift the wholemeal flour, cocoa powder, and baking powder.
2. Then add the brown sugar and mix all the dry ingredients together.
3. Peel bananas and make the pulp.
4. Proceed by mashing the pulp of the bananas with a fork and cut the pear into cubes.
5. Add the liquid ingredients to the powders and mix well until you get a smooth consistency.
6. Add the banana pulp, continuing to mix until the fruit is incorporated into the mixture.

7. Pour everything into a baking pan that you have previously oiled and floured.

8. Bake in a static oven at 190 ºC for about 30 minutes.

9. Always check the cooking, and as soon as it is cooked, let it cool.

10. Slice and serve.

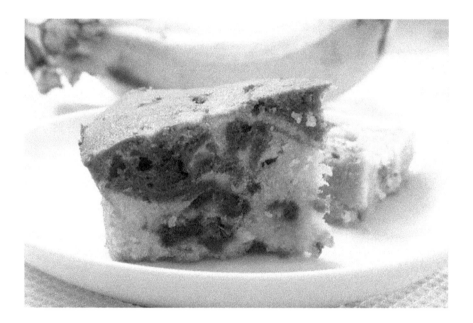

Banana orange and chocolate cake

PREPARATION TIME: 15 minutes
COOKING TIME: 65 minutes
CALORIES: 445

INGREDIENTS FOR 6/8 SERVINGS

- 400 grams of wholemeal flour

- 10 grams of sugar free cocoa powder

- 150 grams of vegan brown sugar

- 250 ml of almond milk

- 1 orange juice

- 120 grams of sunflower oil

- 40 grams of dark vegan chocolate chips

- 1 sachet of natural leavening powder

- 2 ripe bananas

DIRECTIONS

1. First, squeeze the juice from the orange.
2. In a large bowl, sift the wholemeal flour, cocoa powder and baking powder.
3. Then add the brown sugar and mix all the dry ingredients together.
4. Peel bananas and make the pulp.
5. Proceed by mashing the pulp of the bananas with a fork and cut the pear into cubes.

6. Add the liquid ingredients to the powders and mix well until you get a smooth consistency.

7. Add the banana pulp and the chocolate chips, continuing to mix until the fruit is incorporated into the mixture.

8. Pour everything into a baking pan that you have previously oiled and floured.

9. Bake in a static oven at 190 ºC for about 30 minutes.

10. Always check the cooking, and as soon as it is cooked, let it cool.

11. Slice and serve.

Chocolate and rice milk plum cake

PREPARATION TIME: 10 minutes
COOKING TIME: 15/20 minutes
CALORIES: 385

INGREDIENTS FOR 4/5 SERVINGS

- 60 grams of wholemeal flour
- 120 grams of vegan brown sugar
- 200 ml of rice milk
- 3 tablespoons of corn oil
- 8 grams of cream of tartar
- 80 grams of unsweetened sugar free cocoa

DIRECTIONS

1. In a large bowl sift the whole-wheat flour together with the baking powder, and then add the sugar and then the cocoa powder.
2. Mix the powders well together.
3. Now add the liquids: corn oil and rice milk.
4. Mix the mixture with the help of a spoon until it is very homogeneous: it must not be excessively solid / lumpy.
5. Pour the mixture into the plum cake mold.
6. Bake in a preheated static oven at 180 ° C for about 15/20 minutes.
7. Once ready, let the cocoa plum cake cool and serve.

Coconut plum cake

PREPARATION TIME: 10 minutes
COOKING TIME: 15/20 minutes
CALORIES: 356

INGREDIENTS FOR 4/5 SERVINGS

- 100 grams of wholemeal flour
- 40 grams of coconut flour
- 120 grams of vegan brown sugar
- 200 ml of coconut milk
- 1 tablespoon of soy yogurt
- 3 tablespoons of corn oil
- 8 grams of cream of tartar

DIRECTIONS

1. In a large bowl sift the whole-wheat flour together with the baking powder, and then add the sugar and then the coconut flour.
2. Mix the powders well together.
3. Now add the liquids: corn oil, soy yogurt and coconut milk.
4. Mix the mixture with the help of a spoon until it is very homogeneous: it must not be excessively solid / lumpy.
5. Pour the mixture into the plum cake mold.
6. Bake in a preheated static oven at 180 ° C for about 15/20 minutes.
7. Once ready, let the cocoa plum cake cool and serve.

Chocolate and almond plum cake

PREPARATION TIME: 10 minutes
COOKING TIME: 30 minutes
CALORIES: 475

INGREDIENTS FOR 6/8 SERVINGS

- 200 grams of wholemeal flour
- 60 grams of almond flour
- 100 grams of vegan brown sugar
- 20 grams of sugar free cocoa
- 1/2 tablespoon grams of yeast (based on cream of tartar)
- 1 teaspoon of coffee powder
- 60 grams of coconut oil
- 200 grams of almond milk

DIRECTIONS

1. Start the recipe by preparing the dough.
2. In a bowl, pour the wholemeal flour, almond flour, brown sugar, sifted cocoa, coffee and baking powder and mix.
3. Then add the almond milk and coconut oil previously melted in the microwave or in a bain-marie, and mix well with a wooden spoon until the dough is smooth.
4. Line the plum cake mold with parchment paper and pour the mixture into it, then bake in a static oven at 200 ° C for 30 minutes.

5. Test that your cake is cooked by doing the toothpick test: stick it in the centre of the cake and if it comes out dry and without residual dough attached, the plum cake is cooked.

6. Remove from the oven and let it cool completely before serving served sliced.

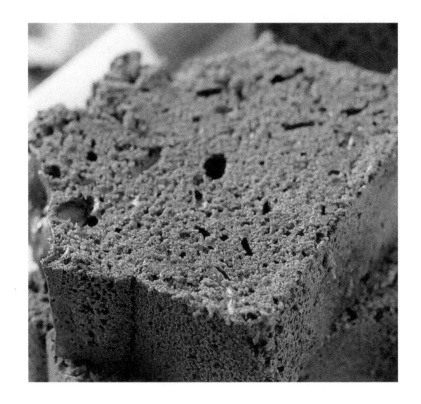

Chocolate and coconut plum cake

PREPARATION TIME: 10 minutes
COOKING TIME: 30 minutes
CALORIES: 490

INGREDIENTS FOR 6/8 SERVINGS

- 200 grams of wholemeal flour
- 60 grams of coconut flour
- 80 grams of vegan brown sugar
- 40 grams of sugar free cocoa
- 200 grams of coconut milk
- 1/2 tablespoon grams of yeast (based on cream of tartar)
- 1 tablespoon of soy yogurt
- 60 grams of coconut oil

DIRECTIONS

1. Start the recipe by preparing the dough.
2. In a bowl, pour the wholemeal flour, coconut flour, brown sugar, sugar free cocoa and baking powder and mix everything together.
3. Then add the coconut milk, soy yogurt, and coconut oil previously melted in the microwave or in a bain-marie, and mix well with a wooden spoon until the dough is smooth.
4. Line the plum cake mold with parchment paper and pour the mixture into it, then bake in a static oven at 200 ° C for 30 minutes.

5. Test that your cake is cooked by doing the toothpick test: stick it in the centre of the cake and if it comes out dry and without residual dough attached, the plum cake is cooked.

6. Remove from the oven and let it cool completely before serving served sliced.

Orange and chocolate plum cake

PREPARATION TIME: 15 minutes
COOKING TIME: 45 minutes
CALORIES: 460

INGREDIENTS FOR 6/8 SERVINGS

- 160 grams of wholemeal flour
- 40 grams of sugar free cocoa
- 50 grams of corn starch
- 100 grams of brown vegan sugar
- 8 grams of natural yeast based on cream of tartar
- 250 grams of natural soy yogurt
- 100 grams of sun flower oil
- 1 orange (zest and juice)
- 30 grams of vegan chocolate chips
- a pinch of baking soda

DIRECTIONS

1. First, prepare the dough.
2. Take a large bowl in which you will put the flour, cocoa powder, corn starch and sugar and yeast.
3. Remember to sift all the dry ingredients so as not to form lumps when you mix everything with the liquids. Grate all the zest of an orange and add the baking soda.
4. Separately create a mixture of soy yogurt, oil and orange juice.

5. Now add the liquid ingredients to the dry ones and mix gently avoiding forming lumps.

6. Finally add chocolate chips and combine well.

7. Prepare the loaf pan: oil and flour it so that the cooking mixture does not stick, or line it with parchment paper. Pour the mixture and bake it at 180 °C in a static oven for 45 minutes.

8. After this time, check the cooking of your plum cake with a toothpick and let it cool.

9. You can serve your orange and chocolate plum cake.

Lemon scented plum cake

PREPARATION TIME: 15 minutes
COOKING TIME: 45 minutes
CALORIES: 380

INGREDIENTS FOR 6/8 SERVINGS

- 200 grams of wholemeal flour
- 50 grams of corn starch
- 100 grams of brown vegan sugar
- 8 grams of natural yeast based on cream of tartar
- 250 grams of natural soy yogurt
- 100 grams of lemon olive oil
- 1 lemon (zest and juice)
- a pinch of baking soda

DIRECTIONS

1. First, prepare the dough.
2. Take a large bowl in which you will put the flour, corn starch and sugar and yeast.
3. Remember to sift all the dry ingredients so as not to form lumps when you mix everything with the liquids. Grate all the zest of a lemon and add the baking soda.
4. Separately create a mixture of soy yogurt, lemon oil and lemon juice.
5. Now add the liquid ingredients to the dry ones and mix gently avoiding forming lumps.

6. Prepare the loaf pan: oil and flour it so that the cooking mixture does not stick, or line it with parchment paper. Pour the mixture and bake it at 180 °C in a static oven for 45 minutes.

7. After this time, check the cooking of your plum cake with a toothpick and let it cool.

8. You can serve your lemon-scented plum cake.

Apple and soy plum cake

PREPARATION TIME: 10 minutes
COOKING TIME: 50 minutes
CALORIES: 315

INGREDIENTS FOR 6/8 SERVINGS

- 150 grams of spelt flour
- 100 grams of wholemeal flour
- 130 g of raw cane vegan sugar
- 10 grams of corn starch
- 1 sachet of natural yeast based on cream of tartar (16 g)
- 125 grams of soy yogurt
- 140 ml of soymilk
- 80 g of sunflower oil
- 1 apple
- ½ lemon
- 1 pinch of salt
- 1 tablespoon of maple syrup
- 1 tablespoon of water

DIRECTIONS

1. In a bowl, combine the 2 flours, vegan cane sugar, corn starch, yeast, and a pinch of salt.
2. Stir with a wooden spoon, and then pour in the soy yogurt, soymilk, sunflower oil and the zest of half a lemon and mix well until you get a homogeneous mixture.

3. In the meantime, wash and peel the apple.

4. Cut half the apple into cubes and add them to the plum cake dough.

5. Then pour the mixture into a lightly greased and floured loaf pan.

6. Slice the other half of the apple and arrange them evenly on the surface of the plum cake, then brush them with maple syrup diluted with water.

7. Bake in a static oven at 180° C for 50 minutes.

8. Remove from the oven, let it cool and gently remove it from the mold. You can enjoy it both warm and after it has cooled completely.

Banana plum cake

PREPARATION TIME: 10 minutes
COOKING TIME: 50 minutes
CALORIES: 315

INGREDIENTS FOR 6/8 SERVINGS

- 250 grams of wholemeal flour
- 130 g of raw cane vegan sugar
- 10 grams of corn starch
- 1 banana
- 1 sachet of natural yeast based on cream of tartar (16 g)
- 125 grams of soy yogurt
- ½ orange
- 140 ml of almond milk
- 80 g of sunflower oil
- 1 pinch of salt

DIRECTIONS

1. In a bowl, combine the wholemeal flour, vegan cane sugar, corn starch, yeast, and a pinch of salt.
2. Stir with a wooden spoon, and then pour in the soy yogurt, almond milk, sunflower oil and the zest of half an orange and mix well until you get a homogeneous mixture.
3. In the meantime, peel and wash the banana.
4. Slice banana and add it to the plum cake dough.
5. Then pour the mixture into a lightly greased and floured loaf pan.

6. Bake in a static oven at 180° C for 50 minutes.

7. Remove from the oven, let it cool and gently remove it from the mold.

8. You can enjoy it both warm and after it has cooled completely.

Vanilla and chocolate little Bundt cakes

PREPARATION TIME: 20 minutes
REST TIME: 2/3 hours
COOKING TIME: 25/30 minutes
CALORIES: 408

INGREDIENTS FOR 10/12 SERVINGS

- 400 grams of wholemeal flour + 2 or 3 tablespoons for kneading *
- 100 grams of sugar free cocoa
- 150 grams of rice milk
- 15 grams of vanilla powder
- 100 grams of vegan brown sugar
- 27 grams of natural yeast
- 150 ml of water
- 60 grams of sunflower oil
- 1 orange zest
- 1 pinch of salt

DIRECTIONS

1. In a large bowl put the flour, cocoa powder, yeast, and sugar and mix well.
2. Add the warm rice milk, water, sunflower oil, salt, vanilla powder, grated orange zest and mix with a spatula.
3. On a work surface add 2 tablespoons of flour and start kneading with your hands.
4. Let the dough absorb all the flour, and then knead vigorously for at least 5 minutes.

5. In the end, your dough needs to be elastic, soft and moist. It should almost stick to the countertop.

6. You can of course use a food processor if you prefer.

7. Brush the inside of a large clean bowl with a little oil.

8. Put the dough on it and brush it with a thin layer of oil. Cover the bowl with a damp kitchen towel and let the dough rise for 2 to 3 hours in a warm place.

9. It needs to at least double in volume, so leave enough space between the dough and the kitchen towel.

10. After rising, transfer the dough to a clean work surface.

11. Fold it in on itself three times then cut it into 9 pieces. Do not use flour here.

12. Take each piece of dough and form a ball.

13. Then with the palm of your hand roll the ball on the work surface to make it smooth and round.

14. Arrange the balls of dough in a lightly oiled mold that can hold all the balls of dough. Let them rest a second time in a warm place for 1 hour.

15. Arranging the vegan dough in a baking pan.

16. Preheat the oven to 180ºC.

17. Place the baking pan in the oven and let cook for 30 minutes about.

18. Once they will be cooked, serve little Bund cakes warm.

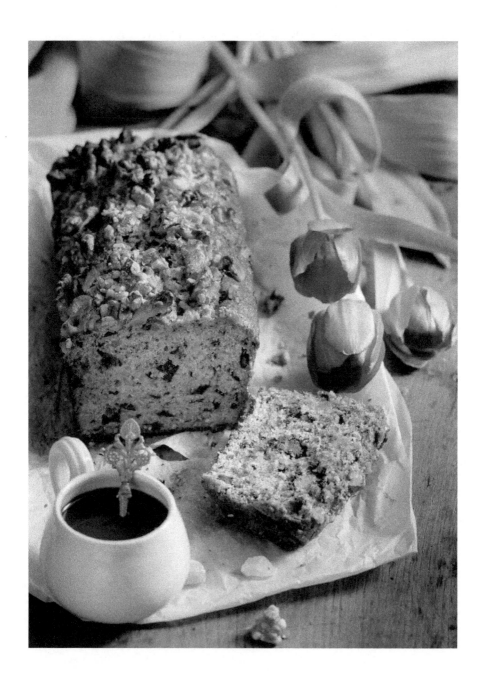

Lime and ginger Bundt cake

PREPARATION TIME: 10 minutes
COOKING TIME: 25 minutes
CALORIES: 300

INGREDIENTS FOR 8 SERVINGS

- 200 grams of wholemeal flour

- 100 g of rice malt

- 120 g of soymilk

- 50 g of sunflower oil

- 1 lemon

- 1 fresh ginger root

- ½ sachet of yeast (cream of tartar)

- 1 pinch of salt

DIRECTIONS

1. Start by preparing the dough
2. Wash the ginger root well and grate it with a grater with small holes.
3. Squeeze the chopped ginger over a small bowl with your hands to collect the juice.
4. Then pour the wholemeal flour, baking powder, lemon zest and salt into a bowl and mix with a wooden spoon.
5. Add the rice malt, sunflower oil, soymilk, lime juice and 4 tablespoons of ginger juice.
6. Mix everything well until you get a homogeneous mixture.
7. Pour the mixture into the previously greased and floured

8. Bundt cake mold.

9. Bake in a static oven at 200 ° C, for 20-25 minutes until the surface of the donut is golden and the inside is cooked.

10. Remove from the oven and let cool completely before serving.

Coconut and almond Bundt cake

PREPARATION TIME: 10 minutes
COOKING TIME: 25 minutes
CALORIES: 300

INGREDIENTS FOR 8 SERVINGS

- 100 grams of wholemeal flour
- 50 grams of almond flour
- 50 grams of coconut flour
- 120 g of almond milk
- 50 ml of coconut oil
- 100 g of rice malt
- 1 lime zest and juice
- ½ sachet of yeast (cream of tartar)
- 1 pinch of salt

DIRECTIONS

1. Start by preparing the dough
2. Pour the wholemeal flour, coconut and almond one, and baking powder, into a bowl. Add lime zest and salt and mix with a wooden spoon.
3. Melt coconut oil in the microwave.
4. Now, add to the powders, rice malt, coconut oil, almond milk, and lime juice-
5. Mix everything well until you get a homogeneous mixture.
6. Pour the mixture into the previously greased and floured

7. Bundt cake mold.

8. Bake in a static oven at 200 ° C, for 20-25 minutes until the surface of the donut is golden and the inside is cooked.

9. Remove from the oven and let cool completely before serving.

Orange and apple Bundt cake

PREPARATION TIME: 15 minutes
COOKING TIME: 30 minutes
CALORIES: 340

INGREDIENTS FOR 8 SERVINGS

- 300 grams of wholemeal flour
- 50 grams of corn starch
- 150 grams of vegan whole cane sugar
- 1 sachet of natural yeast based on cream of tartar
- 1/2 teaspoon of vanilla powder
- 1 pinch of salt
- 100 ml sunflower oil
- 150 ml of soymilk
- 250 g of soy yogurt
- 2 apples
- 1 orange
- sugar-free rolled oats

DIRECTIONS

1. First, grate the orange zest and squeeze it to extract the juice.
2. Peel the apples, core them and cut them into thin slices, perhaps with the help of a mandolin.
3. Put them in a bowl and sprinkle them with the orange juice.
4. Separately in a large bowl, sift the flour, starch and yeast.

5. Add the sugar, a pinch of salt and the grated orange zest.

6. Stir to mix the ingredients well. Now add the soy yogurt, soymilk and sunflower oil.

7. Mix until you get a soft and homogeneous mixture that will be the base of your Bundt cake.

8. Add the sliced apples to the dough and mix them well with the other ingredients.

9. Pour into a previously oiled and floured 22 cm Bundt cake mold, then decorate the surface with the rolled oats and bake in a static oven at 200 ° C for about 30/35 minutes.

10. Before finishing cooking, check the actual cooking of the cake with a toothpick, which could take a few more minutes in the oven depending on the apples chosen.

11. Let cool and serve.

Spelt and apple Bundt cake

PREPARATION TIME: 15 minutes
COOKING TIME: 30 minutes
CALORIES: 386

INGREDIENTS FOR 8 SERVINGS

- 300 grams of wholemeal spelt flour
- 50 grams of potato starch
- 150 grams of vegan whole cane sugar
- 1 lemon
- 1 sachet of natural yeast based on cream of tartar
- 1/2 teaspoon of vanilla powder
- 1 pinch of salt
- 100 ml sunflower oil
- 150 ml of soymilk
- 250 g of soy yogurt
- 2 apples
- Vegan chocolate chips

DIRECTIONS

1. First, grate the lemon zest and squeeze it to extract the juice.
2. Peel the apples, core them and cut them into thin slices, perhaps with the help of a mandolin.
3. Put them in a bowl and sprinkle them with the lemon juice.
4. Separately in a large bowl, sift the spelt flour, potato starch and yeast.
5. Add the sugar, a pinch of salt and the grated orange zest.

6. Stir to mix the ingredients well. Now add the soy yogurt, soymilk and sunflower oil.

7. Mix until you get a soft and homogeneous mixture that will be the base of your Bundt cake.

8. Add the sliced apples to the dough and mix them well with the other ingredients.

9. Pour into a previously oiled and floured 22 cm Bundt cake mold, then decorate the surface with the vegan chocolate chips and bake in a static oven at 200 ° C for about 30/35 minutes.

10. Before finishing cooking, check the actual cooking of the cake with a toothpick, which could take a few more minutes in the oven depending on the apples chosen.

11. Let cool and serve.

Spicy chocolate Bundt cake

PREPARATION TIME: 10 minutes
COOKING TIME: 30 minutes
CALORIES: 380

INGREDIENTS FOR 6/8 SERVINGS

- 150 grams of wholemeal flour

- 100 grams of oat flour

- 250 ml of oat milk

- 100 ml of agave syrup

- 25 grams of sugar free cocoa

- 50 grams of vegan brown sugar

- 60 ml of sunflower oil

- 20 ml of extra virgin olive oil

- 1 teaspoon of chili powder

- 1 sachet of cream of tartar

DIRECTIONS

1. First, sift both flours in a large bowl.

2. Add and sift the yeast and cocoa.

3. Add the sugar and the chilli powder.

4. Separately, mix the liquids, then the two types of oil, oat milk and agave syrup.

5. Combine the dry ingredients with the well-mixed liquid ones and mix everything vigorously avoiding the formation of lumps.

6. Pour the impact into a previously oiled 22 cm diameter Bundt cake pan.

7. Bake at 200 ° C, static oven, for about 30 minutes.

8. As soon as it is cooked, take it out of the oven, cut it and serve.

Corn chocolate Bundt cake

PREPARATION TIME: 10 minutes

COOKING TIME: 30 minutes
CALORIES: 380

INGREDIENTS FOR 6/8 SERVINGS

- 150 grams of wholemeal flour
- 100 grams of corn flour
- 30 grams of sugar free cocoa
- 120 ml of marble syrup
- 250 ml of homemade corn milk (see basic recipe)
- 50 grams of vegan brown sugar
- 60 ml of sunflower oil
- 20 ml of extra virgin olive oil
- 1 teaspoon of vanilla powder
- 1 sachet of cream of tartar

DIRECTIONS

1. First, sift both flours in a large bowl.
2. Add and sift the yeast and cocoa.
3. Add the sugar and the vanilla powder.
4. Separately, mix the liquids, then the two types of oil, corn milk and marble syrup.
5. Combine the dry ingredients with the well-mixed liquid ones and mix everything vigorously avoiding the formation of lumps.
6. Pour the impact into a previously oiled 22 cm diameter Bundt cake pan.

7. Bake at 200 ° C, static oven, for about 30 minutes.

8. As soon as it is cooked, take it out of the oven, cut it and serve.

Double coloured Bundt cake

PREPARATION TIME: 15 minutes
COOKING TIME: 60 minutes
CALORIES: 420

INGREDIENTS FOR 8/10 SERVINGS

- 300 grams of wholemeal flour
- 150 grams of water + 25 grams for the cocoa mixture
- 300 grams of soymilk, soy
- 70 grams of vegan brown sugar
- 40 grams sunflower oil
- 20 grams of sugar free cocoa powder
- 20 grams drops of vegan dark chocolate
- 15 grams of baking powder or cream of tartar
- 1 pinch of vanilla powder
- 1 grated orange zest
- 2 pinches of salt

DIRECTIONS

1. Preheat the oven to 180ºC.
2. Lightly grease a Bundt cake mold, then sprinkle the inside with flour and set aside.
3. In a large bowl, add 150 grams of water.
4. Then add the soymilk, sunflower oil, sugar, vanilla powder, a pinch of salt and mix well.

5. Now sift the flour and baking powder into the bowl with the liquids and mix with a spatula until all the ingredients are combined.

6. Don't mix too much, just time to combine everything.

7. Pour half of the dough into the mold.

8. Halfway through the dough into the mold

9. Add the cocoa powder, dark chocolate chips and 25 grams of water to the remaining dough and mix until the chocolate is evenly distributed.

10. Try not to mix too much.

11. Pour the chocolate mixture into the pan, on top of the white dough.

12. pour the chocolate mixture into the mold

13. Bake in the oven at 180C for 1 hour.

14. Before taking it out, check the inside of the donut with a toothpick. If it comes out dry, the donut is ready.

15. Let it cool, then take it out of the mold, and serve.

Chocolate banana bread

PREPARATION TIME: 15 minutes
COOKING TIME: 40 minutes
CALORIES: 450

INGREDIENTS FOR 6 SERVINGS

- 2 large, very ripe bananas
- 250 grams of wholemeal flour
- 10 grams of oatmeal
- 160 grams of vegan whole cane sugar
- 20 grams of unsweetened sugar free cocoa
- 60 grams of walnuts
- 30 ml of sunflower oil
- 80 ml of almond milk
- 6 tablespoons of boiling water
- 1 teaspoon of vanilla extract
- 5 grams of baking soda
- 1 pinch of salt

DIRECTIONS

1. First, peel and cut the bananas into pieces, or simply take out the pulp.
2. In a bowl, crush the banana pulp well with the help of a fork.
3. Then add the sugar, oil, almond milk and vanilla extract.
4. Open the walnuts and chop them coarsely.
5. Separately, mix the other dry ingredients.

6. Then mix the wholemeal and oat flour with the baking soda and salt, add them to the banana mixture, also pouring the coarsely chopped walnuts with a knife, and mix the minimum necessary to mix the ingredients together.

7. Divide the dough into two equal parts.

8. Dilute the cocoa with 3 tablespoons of boiling water and add it to one-half, while to the mixture that will remain white, add only the other 3 tablespoons of boiling water and mix well.

9. Grease the loaf pan with a drop of oil and sprinkle it with a veil of wholemeal flour.

10. Spoon the two doughs trying to alternate them, and with a long toothpick or the blade of a knife make circular movements to mix the two doughs.

11. Bake in a static oven at 190 ° C for 40 minutes and test the toothpick to make sure the dough is well cooked inside as well.

12. Let the banana bread cool completely before removing it from the mold and serving.

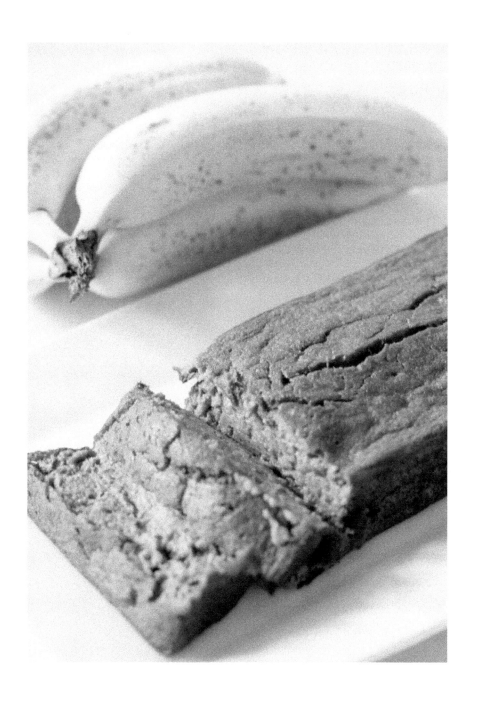

Almond and banana bread

PREPARATION TIME: 15 minutes
COOKING TIME: 40 minutes
CALORIES: 458

INGREDIENTS FOR 6 SERVINGS

- 2 large, very ripe bananas
- 200 grams of wholemeal flour
- 60 grams of corn flour
- 160 grams of vegan whole cane sugar
- 20 grams of unsweetened sugar free cocoa
- 60 grams of almonds
- 30 ml of sunflower oil
- 80 ml of almond milk
- 6 tablespoons of boiling water
- 1 teaspoon of vanilla extract
- 5 grams of baking soda
- 1 pinch of salt

DIRECTIONS

1. First, peel and cut the bananas into pieces, or simply take out the pulp.
2. In a bowl, crush the banana pulp well with the help of a fork.
3. Then add the sugar, oil, almond milk and vanilla extract.
4. Peel and chop almonds very coarsely.
5. Separately, mix the other dry ingredients.

6. Then mix the wholemeal and corn flour with the baking soda and salt, and add them to the banana mixture, also pouring the coarsely chopped almonds with a knife, and mix the minimum necessary to mix the ingredients together.

7. Divide the dough into two equal parts.

8. Dilute the cocoa with 3 tablespoons of boiling water and add it to one-half, while to the mixture that will remain white, add only the other 3 tablespoons of boiling water and mix well.

9. Grease the loaf pan with a drop of oil and sprinkle it with a veil of wholemeal flour.

10. Spoon the two doughs trying to alternate them, and with a long toothpick or the blade of a knife make circular movements to mix the two doughs.

11. Bake in a static oven at 190 ° C for 40 minutes and test the toothpick to make sure the dough is well cooked inside as well.

12. Let the banana bread cool completely before removing it from the mold and serving.

Pistachio and banana bread

PREPARATION TIME: 15 minutes
COOKING TIME: 40 minutes
CALORIES: 490

INGREDIENTS FOR 6 SERVINGS

- 2 large, very ripe bananas

- 200 grams of wholemeal flour

- 60 grams of oat flour

- 160 grams of vegan whole cane sugar

- 20 grams of pistachio homemade cream (see basic recipe)

- 50 grams of pistachios

- 30 ml of sunflower oil

- 80 ml of almond milk

- 1 teaspoon of vanilla extract

- 5 grams of baking soda

- 1 pinch of salt

DIRECTIONS

1. First, peel and cut the bananas into pieces, or simply take out the pulp.

2. In a bowl, crush the banana pulp well with the help of a fork.

3. Then add the sugar, oil, almond milk and vanilla extract.

4. Peel and chop pistachios very coarsely.

5. Separately, mix the other dry ingredients.

6. Then mix the wholemeal and oat flour with the baking soda and salt, add them to the banana mixture, also pouring the coarsely chopped pistachios with a knife, and mix the minimum necessary to mix the ingredients together.

7. Finally add pistachio cream and stir well.

8. Grease the loaf pan with a drop of oil and sprinkle it with a veil of wholemeal flour.

9. Bake in a static oven at 190 ° C for 40 minutes and test the toothpick to make sure the dough is well cooked inside as well.

10. Let the banana pistachio bread cool completely before removing it from the mold and serving.

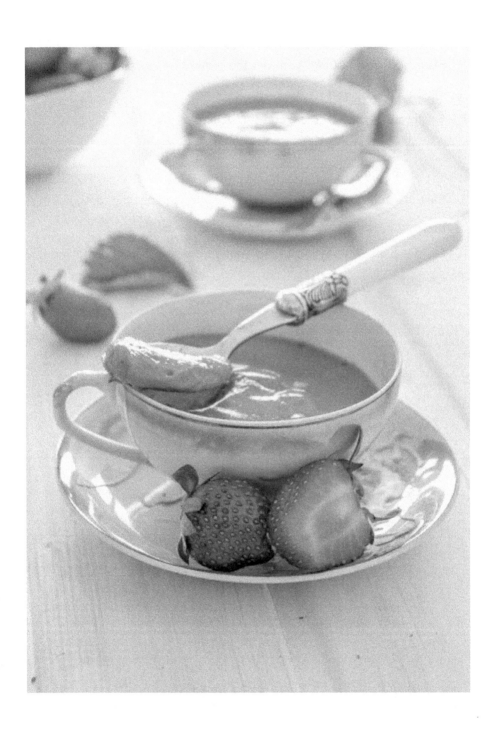

Raspberry and tofu mini parfait

PREPARATION TIME: 10 minutes
REST TIME: 3 hours in the fridge
CALORIES: 160

INGREDIENTS FOR 4 SERVINGS

- 60 ml of olive oil
- 60 grams of coconut oil
- 110 gr of tofu cheese
- 40 grams of vegan cane sugar
- 15 fresh raspberries
- 2 teaspoons of lemon juice

DIRECTIONS

1. First, melt the coconut oil in a low-power microwave safe bowl.
2. Check it every 10-20 seconds and stir it often until it is completely dissolved.
3. cut the tofu into very small pieces
4. In a medium-sized bowl, pour the melted olive oil and coconut oil, add the tofu cheese and mix well.
5. Also, add the sugar, raspberries and lemon juice.
6. Mix all the ingredients well.
7. Pour the mixture into small silicone molds and put them in the freezer for at least 3 hours, until the parfaits have hardened.

8. To serve the mini raspberry parfaits, take them out of the freezer 5 minutes before serving.

9. Remove them from the silicone molds and place them in a small tray, plate or small paper cups.

10. Serve them cold.

Strawberry and almond cheese mini parfait

PREPARATION TIME: 10 minutes
REST TIME: 3 hours in the fridge
CALORIES: 160

INGREDIENTS FOR 4 SERVINGS

- 12 fresh strawberries

- 60 ml of olive oil

- 60 grams of coconut oil

- 120 grams of homemade almond cheese (see basic recipe)

- 40 grams of vegan cane sugar

- 2 teaspoons of orange juice

DIRECTIONS

1. First, melt the coconut oil in a low-power microwave safe bowl.

2. Check it every 10-20 seconds and stir it often until it is completely dissolved.

3. Cut the almond cheese into very small pieces.

4. Wash and remove starch from the strawberries.

5. Meanwhile, squeeze orange juice.

6. In a medium-sized bowl, pour the melted olive oil and coconut oil, add the almond cheese and mix well.

7. Add the sugar, strawberries and orange juice.

8. Mix all the ingredients well.

9. Pour the mixture into small silicone molds and put them in the freezer for at least 3 hours, until the parfaits have hardened.

10. To serve the parfaits, take them out of the freezer 5 minutes before serving.
11. Remove them from the silicone molds and place them in a small tray, plate or small paper cups.
12. Serve them cold.

Marble syrup and raspberry parfait

PREAPARATION TIME: 10 minutes
REST TIME: at least 3 hours in the fridge
CALORIES: 160

INGREDIENTS FOR 4 SERVINGS

- 300 grams of raspberries
- 360 ml of soy yogurt
- 120 ml of soymilk
- 30 grams of vegan brown sugar
- 20 grams of organic honey

DIRECTIONS

1. Firstly, wash the raspberries by passing them quickly under a jet of running water and dry them with a paper towel.
2. Blend them and filter the mixture, passing it through a fine mesh strainer.
3. Combine the raspberry juice, soy yogurt, soymilk, brown sugar and honey in the mixer and stir until the mixture is smooth.
4. Pour it into a parfait molds and freeze them in the freezer for a few hours, preferably overnight.
5. To serve, quickly immerse the molds in warm water and unmold the parfaits.
6. You can serve.

Marble syrup and raspberry parfait

PREAPARATION TIME: 10 minutes
REST TIME: at least 3 hours in the fridge
CALORIES: 160

INGREDIENTS FOR 4 SERVINGS

- 300 grams of raspberries

- 360 ml of soy yogurt

- 120 ml of soymilk

- 30 grams of vegan brown sugar

- 20 grams of marble syrup

DIRECTIONS

1. Firstly, wash the raspberries by passing them quickly under a jet of running water and dry them with a paper towel.

2. Blend them and filter the mixture, passing it through a fine mesh strainer.

3. Combine the raspberry juice, soy yogurt, soymilk, brown sugar and marble syrup in the mixer and stir until the mixture is smooth.

4. Pour it into a parfait molds and freeze them in the freezer for a few hours, preferably overnight.

5. To serve, quickly immerse the molds in warm water and unmold the parfaits.

6. You can serve.

Honey and blueberries parfait

PREAPARATION TIME: 10 minutes
REST TIME: at least 3 hours in the fridge
CALORIES: 160

INGREDIENTS FOR 4 SERVINGS

- 300 grams of blueberries
- 20 grams of (100 % organic) honey
- 360 ml of soy yogurt
- 120 ml of coconut milk
- 30 grams of vegan brown sugar

DIRECTIONS

1. Firstly, wash the blueberries by passing them quickly under a jet of running water and dry them with a paper towel.
2. Blend them and filter the mixture, passing it through a fine mesh strainer.
3. Combine the blueberry juice, soy yogurt, soymilk, brown sugar and honey in the mixer and stir until the mixture is smooth.
4. Pour it into a parfait molds and freeze them in the freezer for a few hours, preferably overnight.
5. To serve, quickly immerse the molds in warm water and unmold the parfaits.
6. You can serve.

Peaches and wild strawberries parfait

PREPATION TIME: 15 minutes
REST TIME: at least 5 hours in the freezer
CALORIES: 180

INGREDIENTS FOR 4 SERVINGS

For the peach compound:
- 2 ripe yellow nectarines

- 50 ml of peach juice

- 125 grams of soy yogurt

- 40 grams of vegan brown sugar

- juice of ½ lemon

- ½ vanilla pod

For the wild strawberry compound:
- 125 grams of wild strawberries

- 40 grams of organic honey

- 125 grams of soy yogurt

- the juice of ½ lemon

- ½ vanilla pod

DIRECTIONS

1. Firstly, cut the nectarines into cubes and collect them in the blender together with the peach and lemon juice, soy yogurt, vanilla seeds and brown sugar.

2. When the mixture is homogeneous, transfer it into a parfait mold filling them up to 1-2 cm from the edge.

3. Place the parfait in the freezer for 30 minutes and the remaining peach cream, already blended, in the refrigerator.

4. Now blend the wild strawberries together with honey, vanilla seeds, and filtered lemon juice and soy yogurt.

5. Divide the wild strawberry mixture into molds pouring it over the peach layer.

6. Stick with ice cream skewers and place in the freezer for about 45 minutes.

7. After this time, remove the first parfait from the freezer and pour the peach cream left over on the wild strawberry mixture.

8. Place again in the freezer for at least 3-4 hours.

9. When serving, gently turn out the two-coloured peach parfait from the molds, helping yourself, only if necessary, with a drizzle of warm running water.

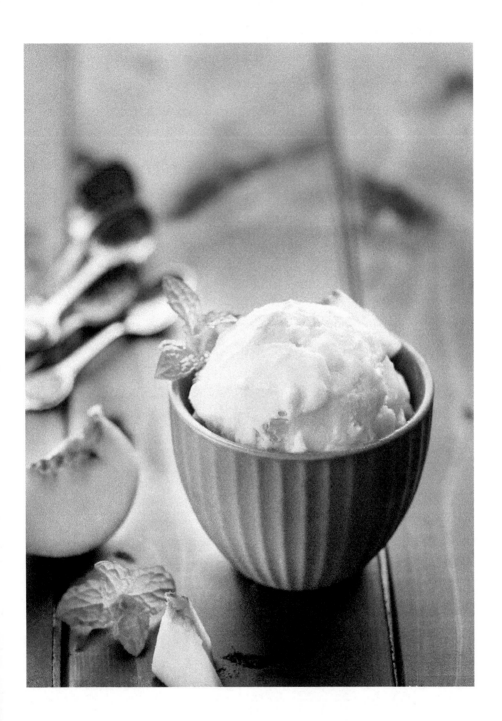

Pears and strawberries vanilla parfait

PREPATION TIME: 15 minutes
REST TIME: at least 5 hours in the freezer
CALORIES: 180

INGREDIENTS FOR 4 SERVINGS

For the pear compound:
- 2 ripe pears

- 50 ml of apple juice

- 125 grams of soy yogurt

- 40 grams of vegan brown sugar

- juice of ½ orange

- ½ vanilla pod

For the strawberry compound:
- 125 grams of strawberries

- 40 grams of organic honey

- 125 grams of soy yogurt

- the juice of ½ orange

- ½ vanilla pod

DIRECTIONS

1. Firstly, peel cut the pears into cubes and collect them in the blender together with the apple and orange juice, soy yogurt, vanilla seeds and brown sugar.

2. When the mixture is homogeneous, transfer it into a parfait mold filling them up to 1-2 cm from the edge.

3. Place the parfait in the freezer for 30 minutes and the remaining peach cream, already blended, in the refrigerator.
4. Now blend the strawberries together with honey, vanilla seeds, filtered orange juice and soy yogurt.
5. Divide the strawberry mixture into molds pouring it over the peach layer.
6. Stick with ice cream skewers and place in the freezer for about 45 minutes.
7. After this time, remove the first parfait from the freezer and pour the peach cream left over on the strawberry mixture.
8. Place again in the freezer for at least 3-4 hours.
9. When serving, gently turn out the two-colored peach parfait from the molds, helping yourself, only if necessary, with a drizzle of warm running water.

Coconut panna cotta

PREPARATION TIME: 2 minutes
COOKING TIME: 15 minutes
REST TIME: 6 hours of rest in the fridge
CALORIES: 190

INGREDIENTS FOR 2 SERVINGS

- 200 ml of soymilk cream

- 8 teaspoons of natural sweetener (stevia)

- 1 tablespoons of powdered agar agar

- 2 tablespoons of coconut flour

DIRECTIONS

1. You can start by putting the soymilk cream and stevia in a saucepan.

2. Heat over low heat, stirring constantly.

3. As soon as the soymilk comes to a boil, remove it from the heat and add the powdered agar agar.

4. Also add the two tablespoons of coconut flour and mix well

5. Stir with a wooden spoon to mix well the gelatine and coconut.

6. Pour the panna cotta into 2 aluminium cups and put it to rest in the fridge for at least 6 hours.

7. As soon as it is time to serve the panna cotta, put very hot water in a container and immerse the bottom of the cups for a few seconds.

8. Then take them and turn them upside down on a serving dish.

9. You can serve with a little coconut flour sprinkled on top (optional).

Coconut and pistachio panna cotta

PREPARATION TIME: 2 minutes
COOKING TIME: 15 minutes
REST TIME: 6 hours of rest in the fridge
CALORIES: 230
INGREDIENTS FOR 2 SERVINGS

- 200 ml of soymilk cream

- 2 tablespoons of coconut flour

- 2 tablespoons of chopped pistachios divided

- 8 teaspoons of natural sweetener (stevia)

- 1 tablespoons of powdered agar agar

DIRECTIONS

1. You can start by putting the soymilk cream and stevia in a saucepan.

2. Heat over low heat, stirring constantly.

3. As soon as the soymilk comes to a boil, remove it from the heat and add the powdered agar agar.

4. Also add the two tablespoons of coconut flour and one tablespoon of pistachio flour and mix well

5. Stir with a wooden spoon to mix well the gelatine and coconut.

6. Pour the panna cotta into 2 aluminium cups and put it to rest in the fridge for at least 6 hours.

7. As soon as it is time to serve the panna cotta, put very hot water in a container and immerse the bottom of the cups for a few seconds.

8. Then take them and turn them upside down on a serving dish.

9. You can serve with a little coconut flour sprinkled on top (optional).

Panna cotta with chocolate

PREPARATION TIME: 10 minutes
COOKING TIME: 10 minutes
REST TIME: 6 hours of rest in the fridge
CALORIES: 180
INGREDIENTS FOR 2 SERVINGS

- 200 ml of unsweetened coconut milk

- 1 teaspoon of agar agar

- 1 tablespoon of sugar free cocoa

- 2 teaspoons of stevia powder

- a vanilla pod

DIRECTIONS

1. You can start by putting the coconut milk in a saucepan along with the stevia.

2. Leave a little milk to one side to mix the gelatine later.

3. Heat over low heat, stirring constantly.

4. As soon as the coconut milk comes to a boil, remove it from the heat and add the agar agar.

5. Also, add cocoa and vanilla and mix well.

6. Pour the panna cotta into 2 aluminium cups and put it to rest in the fridge for at least 6 hours.

7. As soon as it is time to serve the panna cotta, put very hot water in a container and immerse the bottom of the cups for a few seconds.

8. Then take them and turn them upside down on a serving plate.

Vanilla and wild berries panna cotta

PREPARATION TIME: 10 minutes
COOKING TIME: 10 minutes
REST TIME: 1 hour out of the fridge and 5 hours of rest in the fridge
CALORIES: 240

INGREDIENTS FOR 2 SERVINGS

- 250 ml soymilk cream

- 1 teaspoon of vanilla powder

- 60 grams of vegan brown sugar

- 1 teaspoon of agar agar

- 200 grams of wild berries

- 2 tablespoons of vegan brown sugar

DIRECTIONS

1. First, pour the soy cream into a saucepan, add the vanilla powder and the brown sugar.

2. Mix everything well and bring to a boil.

3. As soon as it starts to boil, add the agar agar and continue cooking for 3 minutes.

4. Remove from the heat and with a ladle, pour the mixture into the containers, and let it cool for an hour out of the fridge.

5. Then place the containers in the refrigerator for at least 5 hours.

6. Wash the berries thoroughly and pour them into a bowl with 2 tablespoons of vegan brown sugar, mix them gently so as not to crush them too much and place them in the refrigerator.

7. After the rest time in the refrigerator, remove the panna cotta and turn it out directly on the serving saucer, add a few tablespoons of berries and its sauce created during the marinade.

Almonds panna cotta in raspberry sauce

PREPARATION TIME: 10 minutes
COOKING TIME: 10 minutes
REST TIME: 6 hours of rest in the fridge
CALORIES: 190

INGREDIENTS FOR 2 SERVINGS

For panna cotta:
- 320 grams of almond milk

- 80 grams of peeled almonds soaked for at least an hour

- 12 grams of corn starch

- 4 grams agar agar

- 60 grams of maple syrup

- zest of 1/2 lemon

- 2 teaspoons of vanilla extract

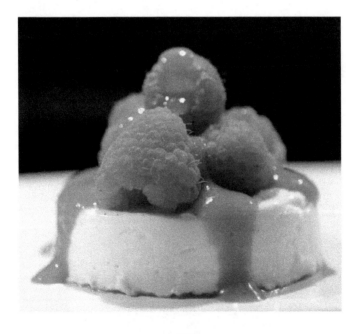

For the raspberry sauce:

- 160 grams fresh raspberries

- 40 grams maple syrup

To serve:

- fresh washed mint

- raspberries

DIRECTIONS

1. Start preparing the raspberry sauce.

2. Wash raspberries under running water and let them dry.

3. In a saucepan, combine the raspberries and maple syrup.

4. Cook over low heat 3-4 minutes and blend with an immersion blender. Continue cooking and let reduce by half.

5. Pass the sauce through a fine mesh colander or gauze to remove the seeds of the raspberries. Let it cool down.

6. Add the almond milk, the drained and rinsed almonds, the maple syrup, the corn starch and the agar agar in the glass of a blender and blend until a homogeneous and smooth cream is obtained.

7. Blend well, if lumps remain it means that the almonds are not well blended. Use a hand blender if necessary.

8. Transfer to a saucepan and bring to a boil.

9. Add the vanilla and lemon zest and simmer for 8-10 minutes.

10. Blend and transfer to the desired container / glass.

11. Let it cool and keep in the fridge for at least 6/8 hours or overnight.

12. The next day, serve the panna cotta with the warm or cold raspberry sauce, fresh raspberries and sprigs of mint.

Raspberries and peaches frozen soy yogurt

PREPATION TIME: 40 minutes
REST TIME: at least 4 hours in the freezer
CALORIES: 170

INGREDIENTS FOR 4 SERVINGS

- 250 grams of raspberries
- 2 yellow-fleshed peaches
- 600 grams of soy yogurt
- 130 grams of vegan brown sugar

DIRECTIONS

1. Start washing raspberries.
2. Take 200 grams of them setting the remaining 50 grams aside.
3. Cook 200 grams of raspberries with half the brown sugar and a couple of tablespoons of water.
4. When the berries are soft, pass them through a colander, crushing them with a spoon to make the pulp come out well.
5. Set aside 2-3 tablespoons of pulp in a small glass that you will need for the final decoration.
6. Now, peel and slice peaches.
7. In the same way of raspberries, cook the sliced peaches with the second half of the sugar and two tablespoons of water.
8. When cooked, reduce to cream with an immersion beater.

9. Now prepare three bowls: one will contain the peach cream, a second little raspberry cream (2-3 tablespoons) the third all the remaining raspberry pulp.

10. Divide the soy yogurt into 3 parts and add each individual part to the various bowls, whip the cream and pour it into the three bowls.

11. With a spatula, gently mix the ingredients.

12. In this way, you will get 3 different shades of colour.

13. In a pudding mold, pour the first part of the raspberry cream, the darker one.

14. Place the mold in the freezer for 5-6 minutes, then remove the mold and pour in the lighter raspberry cream. Leave to rest in the freezer again and then complete with the peach cream. Leave to rest in the freezer for another 3-4 hours.

15. Take the frozen yogurt 10 minutes before serving. Complete with the 50 grams of raspberries kept aside and a few tablespoons of raspberry pulp.

Strawberries and banana frozen soy yogurt

PREPATION TIME: 40 minutes
REST TIME: at least 4 hours in the freezer
CALORIES: 215

INGREDIENTS FOR 4 SERVINGS

- 300 grams of strawberries

- 1 ripe banana

- 600 grams of soy yogurt

- 130 grams of vegan brown sugar

DIRECTIONS

1. Start washing strawberries.

2. Clean them removing stalks.

3. Take 250 grams of them setting the remaining 50 grams aside.

4. Cook 250 grams of strawberries with half the brown sugar and a couple of tablespoons of water.

5. When the berries are soft, pass them through a colander, crushing them with a spoon to make the pulp come out well.

6. Set aside 2-3 tablespoons of pulp in a small glass that you will need for the final decoration.

7. Now, peel and slice banana.

8. In the same way of strawberries, cook the sliced banana with the second half of the sugar and two tablespoons of water.

9. When cooked, reduce to cream with an immersion beater.

10. Now prepare three bowls: one will contain the peach cream, a second little strawberry cream (2-3 tablespoons) the third all the remaining strawberry pulp.

11. Divide the soy yogurt into 3 parts and add each individual part to the various bowls, whip the cream and pour it into the three bowls.

12. With a spatula, gently mix the ingredients.

13. In this way, you will get 3 different shades of colour.

14. In a pudding mold, pour the first part of the strawberry cream, the darker one.

15. Place the mold in the freezer for 5-6 minutes, then remove the mold and pour in the lighter strawberry cream.

16. Leave to rest in the freezer again and then complete with the banana cream. Leave to rest in the freezer for another 3-4 hours.

17. Take the frozen yogurt 10 minutes before serving. Complete with the 50 grams of strawberries kept aside and a few tablespoons of strawberry pulp.

Almond milk and raspberries ice cream

PREPATION TIME: 10 minutes
REST TIME: 4 hours in the freezer
CALORIES: 180

INGREDIENTS FOR 4 SERVINGS

- 30 ml of sugar free almond milk
- 20 ml of soymilk whipped cream
- 80 grams of vegan brown sugar
- 300 grams of raspberries

DIRETCIONS

1. Firstly, quickly rinse the raspberries in cold water, drain and lay them out to dry on a paper towel.
2. Blend the almond milk with the raspberries and the brown sugar in a blender until the mixture is homogeneous, and filter it through a fine mesh strainer to eliminate the seeds.
3. Add the soymilk whipped cream, mix and pour the mixture into the ice cream molds. Place the stick in the centre and freeze in the freezer for at least 4 hours.
4. Turn out the ice cream and serve.

Peach ice cream

PREPATION TIME: 10 minutes
REST TIME: 4 hours in the freezer
CALORIES: 180

INGREDIENTS FOR 4 SERVINGS

- 30 ml of almond milk
- 20 ml of soymilk whipped cream
- 80 grams of vegan brown sugar
- 1 ripe peach

DIRETCIONS

1. Firstly, peel and remove stone from the peach.
2. Then, slice it. Rinse the peach pieces in cold water, drain and lay them out to dry on a paper towel.
3. Blend the almond milk with the peach pieces and the brown sugar in a blender until the mixture is homogeneous, and filter it through a fine mesh strainer to eliminate the seeds.
4. Add the soymilk whipped cream, mix and pour the mixture into the ice cream molds.
5. Place the stick in the centre and freeze in the freezer for at least 4 hours.
6. Turn out the ice cream and serve.

Coconut milk and wild strawberries ice cream

PREPATION TIME: 10 minutes
REST TIME: 4 hours in the freezer
CALORIES: 180

INGREDIENTS FOR 4 SERVINGS

- 30 ml of coconut milk
- 300 grams of wild strawberries
- 20 ml of soymilk whipped cream
- 80 grams of vegan brown sugar

DIRETCIONS

1. Firstly, quickly rinse the wild strawberries in cold water, drain and lay them out to dry on a paper towel.

2. Blend the coconut milk with the raspberries and the brown sugar in a blender until the mixture is homogeneous, and filter it through a fine mesh strainer to eliminate the seeds.

3. Add the soymilk whipped cream, mix and pour the mixture into the ice cream molds. Place the stick in the centre and freeze in the freezer for at least 4 hours.

4. Turn out the ice cream and serve.

Strawberry mousse

PREPATION TIME: 20 minutes
COOK TIME: 2 minutes
REST TIME: 1 hour in the fridge
CALORIES: 150

INGREDIENTS FOR 4 SERVINGS

- 250 grams of strawberries
- 60 grams of vegan brown sugar
- 400 ml of soymilk whipped cream
- 4 grams of agar agar powder
- 10-12 fresh strawberries for decoration

DIRECTIONS

1. To prepare the strawberry mousse, first wash the strawberries, removing the stalk, and blend them with an immersion blender, until the mixture is smooth.
2. Add agar agar powder to the strawberry mixture and stir to mix.
3. Whip the soymilk cream with an electric mixer in a clean bowl and incorporate it several times, stirring from the bottom up, to the strawberry mixture.
4. When you have obtained a homogeneous mixture, divide it into the chosen glasses.
5. Refrigerate for 1 hour before serving.
6. At the time of serving, the strawberry mousse completed with diced strawberries.

Strawberry and chocolate mousse

PREPATION TIME: 20 minutes
COOK TIME: 2 minutes
REST TIME: 1 hour in the fridge
CALORIES: 190

INGREDIENTS FOR 4 SERVINGS

- 250 grams of strawberries
- 40 grams of vegan brown sugar
- 20 grams of sugar free cocoa powder
- 1 pinch of vanilla powder
- 400 ml of soymilk whipped cream
- 4 grams of agar agar powder
- 10-12 fresh strawberries for decoration

DIRECTIONS

1. To prepare the strawberry mousse, first clean the strawberries, removing the stalk, and blend them with an immersion blender together with vanilla powder, until the mixture is smooth.
2. Add agar agar and cocoa powder to the strawberry mixture and stir to mix.
3. Whip the soymilk cream with an electric mixer in a clean bowl and incorporate it several times, stirring from the bottom up, to the strawberry mixture.
4. When you have obtained a homogeneous mixture, divide it into the chosen glasses.

5. Refrigerate for 1 hour before serving.

6. At the time of serving the chocolate strawberry mousse completed with diced strawberries.

Raspberry and almond mousse

PREPATION TIME: 20 minutes
COOK TIME: 2 minutes
REST TIME: 1 hour in the fridge
CALORIES: 178

INGREDIENTS FOR 4 SERVINGS

- 250 grams of raspberries
- 60 grams of vegan brown sugar
- 380 ml of soymilk whipped cream
- 20 ml of almond milk
- 4 grams of agar agar powder
- 10-12 almond slices for decoration

DIRECTIONS

1. First clean the raspberries, and blend them with an immersion blender, until the mixture is smooth.
2. Add agar agar powder and almond milk to the strawberry mixture and stir to mix.
3. Whip the soymilk cream with an electric mixer in a clean bowl and incorporate it several times, stirring from the bottom up, to the strawberry mixture.
4. When you have obtained a homogeneous mixture, divide it into the chosen glasses.

5. Refrigerate for 1 hour before serving.

6. At the time of serving the almond raspberry mousse completed with sliced almonds, pour over.

Chocolate and tofu mousse

PREPARATION TIME: 20 minutes
REST TIME: 60 minutes in the fridge
CALORIES: 300

INGREDIENTS FOR 4 SERVINGS

- 200 grams of tofu

- 200 ml of soy whipping cream

- 1 teaspoon of vanilla extract

- 60 grams of unsweetened cocoa powder

- 60 g of stevia powder

- A pinch of salt

DIRECTIONS

1. Take a bowl and put the tofu inside.

2. With an electric mixer, start working the tofu cheese until you have obtained a light and fluffy cream.

3. Set the mixer to minimum speed and add the vanilla extract first and then the soy cream.

4. While continuing to mix, add the sweetener and stir until well blended.

5. Now add the cocoa powder and a pinch of salt, increase the speed of the mixer to the maximum and continue to mix for another 2 minutes, or in any case until you have obtained a soft and homogeneous mixture.

6. Put the mousse to rest in the fridge for an hour and then serve it in four glasses.

Almond cheese and chocolate mousse

PREPARATION TIME: 20 minutes
REST TIME: 60 minutes in the fridge
CALORIES: 345

INGREDIENTS FOR 4 SERVINGS

- 200 grams of homemade almond cheese (see basic recipe)
- 80 grams of unsweetened cocoa powder
- 60 ml of marble syrup
- 200 ml of soy whipping cream
- 1 teaspoon of vanilla extract
- A pinch of salt

DIRECTIONS

1. Take a bowl and put the almond cheese inside.
2. With an electric mixer, start working the cheese until you have obtained a light and fluffy cream.
3. Set the mixer to minimum speed and add the vanilla extract first and then the soy cream.
4. While continuing to mix, add the marble syrup and stir until well blended.
5. Now, add the cocoa powder and a pinch of salt increase the speed of the mixer to the maximum and continue to mix for another 2 minutes or in any case until you have obtained a soft and homogeneous mixture.
6. Put the mousse to rest in the fridge for an hour and then serve it in four glasses

Canadian apples

PREPATION TIME: 15 minutes
COOK TIME: 30 minutes
CALORIES: 160
INGREDIENTS FOR 4 SERVINGS

- 4 large apples

- 80 grams of soy butter

- 70 grams of vegan cane sugar

- A tablespoon of wholemeal flour

- Salt to taste

- 50 grams of shelled walnuts

- 200 grams of soymilk cream

DIRECTIONS

1. Shell the apples, cut them in half and core them, lightly scooping each half apple with a teaspoon.

2. Oil a baking dish and arrange the apples, with the rounded part resting on the bottom of the container.

3. Put the soy butter in a bowl, together with the vegan cane sugar, the wholemeal and a pinch of salt. Work the ingredients for a long time, until you get a soft and fluffy cream.

4. Chop the walnuts and add them to the cream.

5. Now, divide the mixture into eight parts and distribute it in the apple halves.

6. Place in the oven at 200ºC and cook for 30 minutes.

7. Take the apples out of the oven and serve them hot, accompanying them with the liquid soymilk cream.

8. If you want you can also serve this dessert cold.

Apple donuts

PREPATION TIME: 15 minutes
COOK TIME: 15 minutes
REST TIME: at least 1 hour in the fridge
CALORIES: 190

INGREDIENTS FOR 4/5 SERVINGS

- 200 grams of wholemeal flour
- 3 apples
- 150 ml of apple juice
- 110 ml of oat milk
- 20 grams of vegan brown sugar
- ½ teaspoon of natural yeast based on cream of tartar
- Zest of one orange
- 1 pinch of salt
- 1 l peanut oil
- Vegan brown sugar to taste
- Cinnamon to taste

DIRECTIONS

1. First, prepare the batter.
2. In a bowl, pour the wholemeal flour, sugar, baking powder, pinch of salt and orange zest.
3. Stir with a wooden spoon, and then add the apple juice and oat milk.
4. Mix everything well until you get a thick batter.
5. Cover the bowl with plastic wrap and let the batter rest in the refrigerator for at least an hour.

6. in the meantime, peel the apples, remove the stalk and cut them into discs.

7. With the help of a pointed knife, remove the central core from each disc, in order to obtain a sort of apple donut.

8. Heat up the peanut oil in a pan with high sides suitable for frying.

9. To check that the oil has reached the right temperature for frying, pour half a teaspoon of batter into the oil: it must rise from the bottom of the pan to the surface within a few seconds and fry gently.

10. At this point, pass a couple of apple donuts into the dough, drain the excess batter and carefully introduce them into the boiling oil.

11. Let them fry for a few minutes, turning them every now and then with a frying spider so that they brown evenly.

12. When they are swollen and golden, drain them on a tray covered with paper towel. Proceed in this way until all the ingredients are used up.

13. If you like, you can sprinkle the surface of the still hot apple donuts with a little vegan brown sugar and cinnamon.

14. Serve when they are still hot or at most lukewarm.

Vanilla donuts

PREPARATION TIME: 20 minutes
REST TIME: 2/3 hours
COOKING TIME: 25/30 minutes
CALORIES: 325

INGREDIENTS FOR 10/12 SERVINGS

- 500 grams of wholemeal flour + 2 or 3 tablespoons for kneading *
- 100 grams of vegan brown sugar
- 27 grams of natural yeast
- 150 grams of soymilk
- 150 ml of water
- 60 grams of sunflower oil
- 1 vial of vanilla flavour
- 1 orange zest
- 1 pinch of salt

DIRECTIONS

1. In a large bowl put the flour, yeast, and sugar and mix well.
2. Add the warm soymilk, water, and sunflower oil, salt, vanilla, grated orange zest and mix with a spatula.
3. On a work surface add 2 tablespoons of flour and start kneading with your hands.
4. Let the dough absorb all the flour, and then knead vigorously for at least 5 minutes.

5. In the end, your dough needs to be elastic, soft and moist. It should almost stick to the countertop.

6. You can of course use a food processor if you prefer.

7. Brush the inside of a large clean bowl with a little oil.

8. Put the dough on it and brush it with a thin layer of oil. Cover the bowl with a damp kitchen towel and let the dough rise for 2 to 3 hours in a warm place.

9. It needs to at least double in volume, so leave enough space between the dough and the kitchen towel.

10. After rising, transfer the dough to a clean work surface.

11. Fold it in on itself three times then cut it into 9 pieces. Do not use flour here.

12. Take each piece of dough and form a ball.

13. Then with the palm of your hand roll the ball on the work surface to make it smooth and round.

14. Arrange the balls of dough in a lightly oiled mold that can hold all the balls of dough. Let them rest a second time in a warm place for 1 hour.

15. Preheat the oven to 180ºC.

16. Just before baking, brush the top of the balls of dough with soymilk and cook on the lower rack of the oven for about 25-30 minutes.

17. The donuts should be golden on top but still very soft on the inside.

18. Let it cool a bit before sprinkling with icing sugar, peel off a ball and eat it like this, with your hands.

Corn flour and cinnamon donuts

PREPARATION TIME: 20 minutes
COOKING TIME: 30 minutes
CALORIES: 425

INGREDIENTS FOR 4 SERVINGS

- 150 grams of corn flour

- 100 grams of wholemeal flour

- 1 teaspoon of powder cinnamon

- 50 grams of vegan cane sugar

- 20 ml of olive oil

- 1 teaspoon of natural baking powder

- 50 ml of soymilk

DIRECTIONS

1. Put the two flours, brown sugar, cinnamon and yeast in a bowl and mix.

2. Now add the olive oil.

3. Mix and mix everything and then start kneading the mixture with your hands.

4. Add the soymilk and knead until you have obtained a firm and homogeneous mixture.

5. Take 4 donut molds and brush them with a little olive oil.

6. Put a piece of dough inside each mold, levelling it well with your hands.

7. Let them cook at 190º C for 30 minutes.

8. Always check the cooking and if they seem not yet cooked, continue for another couple of minutes.
9. As soon as they are cooked, remove them from the oven and let them cool for 5 minutes.
10. You can serve your donuts.

Corn flour and chocolate donuts

PREPARATION TIME: 20 minutes
COOKING TIME: 30 minutes
CALORIES: 425

INGREDIENTS FOR 4 SERVINGS

- 120 grams of corn flour

- 30 grams of sugar free coco powder

- 100 grams of wholemeal flour

- 1 teaspoon of powder vanilla

- 50 grams of vegan cane sugar

- 20 ml of olive oil

- 1 teaspoon of natural baking powder

- 50 ml of soymilk

DIRECTIONS

11. Put the two flours, brown sugar, vanilla, cocoa powder, and yeast in a bowl and mix.
12. Now add the olive oil.
13. Mix and mix everything and then start kneading the mixture with your hands.
14. Add the soymilk and knead until you have obtained a firm and homogeneous mixture.
15. Take 4 donut molds and brush them with a little olive oil.
16. Put a piece of dough inside each mold, levelling it well with your hands.
17. Let them cook at 190º C for 30 minutes.

18. Always check the cooking and if they seem not yet cooked, continue for another couple of minutes.
19. As soon as they are cooked, remove them from the oven and let them cool for 5 minutes.
20. You can serve your donuts.

Spelt and coconut donuts

PREPARATION TIME: 20 minutes
COOKING TIME: 30 minutes
CALORIES: 425

INGREDIENTS FOR 4 SERVINGS

- 150 grams of spelt flour

- 80 grams of wholemeal flour

- 20 grams of coconut flour

- 50 ml of coconut milk

- 1 teaspoon of powder vanilla

- 50 grams of vegan cane sugar

- 20 ml of olive oil

- 1 teaspoon of natural baking powder

DIRECTIONS

21. Put the 3 flours, brown sugar, vanilla and yeast in a bowl and mix.

22. Now add the olive oil.

23. Mix and mix everything and then start kneading the mixture with your hands.

24. Add the soymilk and knead until you have obtained a firm and homogeneous mixture.

25. Take 4 donut molds and brush them with a little olive oil.

26. Put a piece of dough inside each mold, levelling it well with your hands.

27. Let them cook at 190º C for 30 minutes.

28. Always check the cooking and if they seem not yet cooked, continue for another couple of minutes.
29. As soon as they are cooked, remove them from the oven and let them cool for 5 minutes.
30. You can serve your donuts.

A simple recipe book of desserts to always keep at hand for your best recipes!

I love you, your Carolyn ☺

Plant-Based Dessert

Super tasty vegetable and
Fruit Based Dessert
recipes to lose weight with taste!

Carolyn J Perez

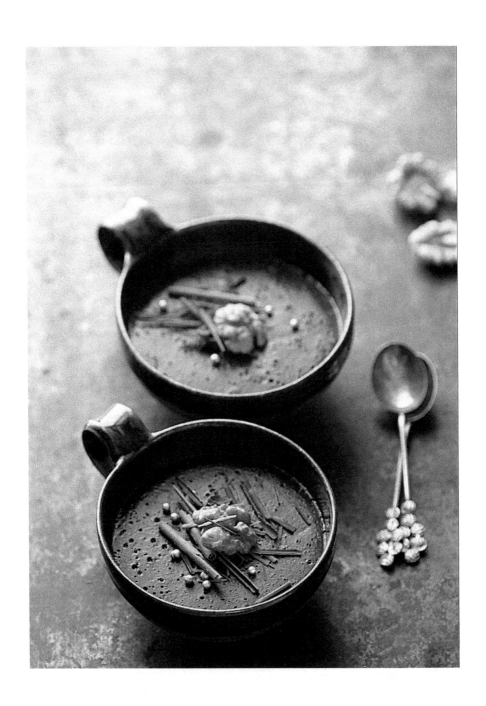

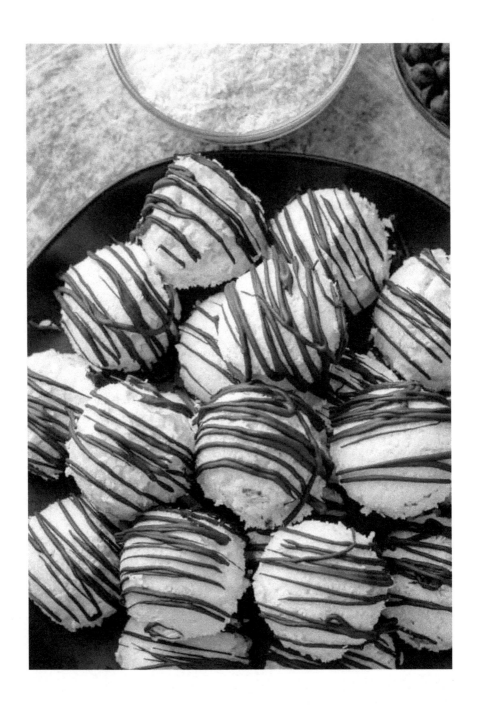

Contents

Introduction

It is a common thought to think that following a diet is necessarily linked to the concept of actual weight loss. However, this is not always the case: following a diet is often directly linked to the foods that we decide to include in our tables daily.

In addition, we do not always choose the best quality ingredients to cook our dishes.

Sometimes we are so rushed and unruly that we forget that we love our bodies. And what better cure than a healthy diet? Following a healthy diet should become more than an imposition or a punishment, but a real lifestyle.

Moreover, this is the Plant-based diet goal: not to impose a restrictive and sometimes impossible diet to follow, but to recreate a diet based on foods of natural origin and above all healthy. Therefore, the plant based represents a real food trend. However, as we will see it is much more than just a fashion trend, but a real lifestyle.

In addition, it is the aim of this text, or rather of this cookbook, to introduce you to the plant based discipline. And we will do it with a few theoretical explanations, just to make you understand what we are talking about and above all how to prepare it: there will be a purely practical part where you will find 800 recipes on the plant based. These recipes will be divided into appetizers, snacks, first and second courses, side dishes and finally a string of plant based desserts.

In the end, you will be spoiled for choice to start following this healthy dietary discipline.

Plant based diet: what are we talking about?

We already mentioned that more than a real weight loss diet the Plant based diet is a food discipline. Food discipline is enjoying great success not only because it is very fashionable, but because it applies such principles that can be perfectly integrated into our daily lives. The plant-based diet is a true approach to life, starting with nutrition: respect for one's health and body, first of all, which is reflected in respect for all forms of life and the planet in general.

As the word itself says, it deals with a food plan based, precisely on what comes from plants. However, simply calling it that way would be too simplistic.

It is a predominantly plant-based diet, but not only. It is not just about consuming vegetables but about taking natural foods: not industrially processed, not treated, and not deriving from the exploitation of resources and animals, preferably zero km.

So it could be a discipline that aims not only at environmental saving but also at the economic one: think about what advantages, in fact, at the level of your pockets you can have if you apply the principle of 0Km and therefore to be able to harvest your vegetables directly from your garden.

Environmental savings do not only mean pollution reduction: the ethical component (present exclusively in the vegan diet, for example) is combined with a strong will to health. This means that the plant based, in addition to not preferring foods that exploit animals, is also based on foods that are especially unprocessed, fresh, healthy, balanced, light, and rich in essential nutrients. In practice, it is a plant-based diet but not vegan / vegetarian, emphasizing the quality and wholesomeness of foods rather than on their moral value, albeit with great attention to sustainability. Such a lifestyle could therefore be of help, not only to our health, but also to create a more sustainable world for future generations.

Main differences between Vegan and Plant based diet

The plant-based diet is often associated with the vegan diet. This is because both plan to include cruelty free foods that do not involve any animal exploitation.

Furthermore, they are associated precisely because they are both predominantly plant-based.

However, there are some pretty obvious differences between these two diets.

First of all, precisely for the reasoning behind the prevalence of plants.

It is well known that even the vegan diet provides a diet based on foods of plant origin: unlike the plant-based diet, however, nothing of animal derivation is allowed, neither direct nor indirect, nor other products - clothing or accessories - which include the exploitation of animals.

No eggs, no milk, no honey, no leather, so to speak, and not only: in its most rigorous meanings, veganism does not even include the use of yeasts, as the bacteria that compose them are indisputably living beings.

A vegan diet can be balanced if the person who leads it knows well the foods and their combinations, the necessary supplements, and their body's reaction to the lack of certain foods.

On the contrary, the Plant-Based diet is on the one hand more relaxed, on the other more stringent.

What does it mean?

This means that it is on the one hand more relaxed because it is plant-based, but not exclusively vegetable: products of animal origin are allowed, in moderate quantities, but under only one condition, namely the excellent quality of the food itself and its certified origin. For example, eggs can be consumed occasionally but only if very fresh, possibly at zero km, from free-range farms where the hens are not exploited but can live outdoors without constraints.

It is also a somewhat more stringent philosophy than veganism precisely for this reason: as long as it is 100% vegetable, the vegan also consumes heavily processed foods, such as industrial fries. Therefore, the vegan can also eat junk foods or snacks. Conversely, plant-based dieters would never admit highly refined foods of this type.

Both dietary approaches are conscious and do not involve the consumption of meat. However, if vegans are driven by ethical reasons, those who follow a plant-based diet also reject everything processed on an industrial level and unhealthy.

A plant-based diet is a diet that aims to eliminate industrially processed foods and, therefore, potentially more harmful to health. It is based on the consumption of fruit and vegetables, whole grains and avoiding (or minimizing) animal products and processed foods. This means that vegan desserts made with refined sugar or bleached flour are also covered.

There is also a substantial difference between the philosophies behind the two diets. As we said in the previous paragraph and above, the ethical component, which is based on the refusal of any food of animal origin, plays a lot in veganism. While for the plant based is not a purely moral and moralistic discourse but on the real thought of being able to keep healthy with the food discipline and be respectful of the environment surrounding us.

Plant based diet full shopping list. What to eat and what to avoid

Now we can examine the complete shopping list of the plant based diet.

Let's briefly summarize the principles on which this particular type of diet is based:

- Emphasizes whole, minimally processed foods.

- Limits or avoids animal products.

- Focuses on plants, including vegetables, fruits, whole grains, legumes, seeds and nuts, which should make up most of what you eat.

- Excludes refined foods, like added sugars, white flour and processed oils.

- Pays special attention to food quality, promoting locally sourced, organic food whenever possible.

As for what you can usually eat, we can say the general consumption of:

- Wholegrain and flours

- extra virgin olive oil

- Seasonal fruit and vegetables: these foods are the basis of every meal.

- In this diet you can also eat sweets but only and exclusively homemade and with controlled raw materials, simple and not very refined, preferably of vegetable origin - for example by replacing milk with soy or rice drinks, and eggs with other natural thickeners such as flaxseed, or simple ripe banana.

- You can also consume nuts and seeds.

As for absolutely forbidden foods, there are all those ready-made and processed:

- ready-made sauces
- chips
- biscuits
- various kinds of snacks
- sugary cereals,
- Spreads, snacks and many other notoriously unhealthy foods.
- Junk food and fast food are therefore absolutely banned
- Sugar beverages

Regarding the complete shopping list:

- Fruits: Berries, citrus fruits, pears, peaches, pineapple, bananas, etc.

- Vegetables: Kale, spinach, tomatoes, broccoli, cauliflower, carrots, asparagus, peppers, etc.

- Starchy vegetables: Potatoes, sweet potatoes, butternut squash, etc.

- Whole grains: Brown rice, rolled oats, spelt, quinoa, brown rice pasta, barley, etc.

- Healthy fats with omega 3: Avocados, olive oil, coconut oil, unsweetened coconut, etc.

- Legumes: Peas, chickpeas, lentils, peanuts, beans, black beans, etc.

- Seeds, nuts and nut butter: Almonds, cashews, macadamia nuts, pumpkin seeds, sunflower seeds, natural peanut butter, tahini, etc.

- Unsweetened plant-based milk: Coconut milk, almond milk, cashew milk, etc.

- Spices, herbs and seasonings: Basil, rosemary, turmeric, curry, black pepper, salt, etc.

- Condiments: Salsa, mustard, nutritional yeast, soy sauce, vinegar, lemon juice, etc.

- Plant-based protein: Tofu, tempeh, seitan, and plant based protein sources or powders with no added sugar or artificial ingredients.
- Beverages: Coffee, tea, sparkling water, etc.

There is the chance to add food of animal origin very rarely, for example if you have specific nutritional needs or if it has been strongly recommended by your doctor. Anyway, if supplementing your plant-based diet with animal products choose quality products from grocery stores or, better yet, purchase them from local farms.

- Eggs: Pasture-raised when possible.
- Poultry: Free-range, organic when possible.
- Beef and pork: Pastured or grass-fed when possible.
- Seafood: Wild-caught from sustainable fisheries when possible.
- Dairy: Organic dairy products from pasture-raised animals whenever possible.

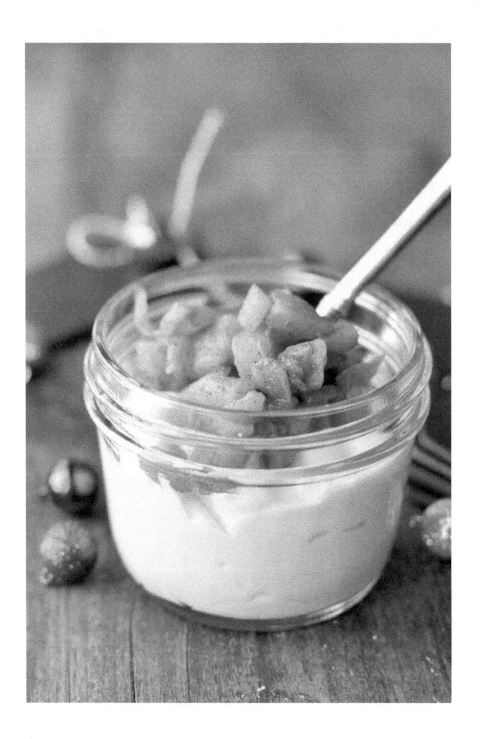

Dessert and fruit recipes

Strawberry crepes

PREPARATION TIME: 15 minutes
COOKING TIME: 10 minutes
CALORIES: 210

NGREDIENTS FOR 2/3 SERVINGS

- 140 gram of wholemeal flour

- 300 ml of soymilk

- 40 grams of wholemeal vegan brown sugar

- 1 teaspoon of extra virgin olive oil

For the filling:

- 12 strawberries

- 1 vanilla pod

- 20 ml of marble syrup

- 150 ml of water

DIRECTIONS

1. Start preparing crepes dough.

2. In a bowl pour the wholemeal flour and vegan brown sugar, mix with a spoon to mix the dry ingredients.

3. At this point, add the soymilk and with the help of a whisk, mix everything until the mixture is liquid and uniform.

4. Depending on the wholemeal flour used - which can absorb more or less liquids - you may have to add a little more milk.

5. Now you can prepare the filling

6. Separately, boil the water in which you have put the marble syrup and the vanilla pod: let it simmer for a few minutes to prepare your infusion.

7. Meanwhile, take strawberries, wash them, remove the stalk and cut them into 4 and put them in the pan.

8. Turn on the heat over medium heat and sprinkle with your vanilla infusion, remembering to stir from time to time.

9. Your strawberry filling will be ready when all the water has dried (about 10 minutes).

10. Now, cook crepes.

11. Grease a non-stick pan with a veil of oil, eliminating any excess with a paper towel.

12. Put it on the fire, let it heat well for 1 minute: now you can pour a ladle of mixture in the centre.

13. For a pan with a diameter of 20 cm, it will be the right amount to get your crepe not too thick.

14. Let it cook for about a minute on each side, then remove it from the heat and place it on a cutting board: continue with the process until the dough is finished, placing the crepes on top of each other so that they keep well moist.

15. Fill your crepes with the strawberry filling and serve.

Nutella crepes

PREPARATION TIME: 15 minutes

COOKING TIME: 10 minutes
CALORIES: 305

NGREDIENTS FOR 2/3 SERVINGS

- 140 gram of wholemeal flour

- 300 ml of soymilk

- 40 grams of wholemeal vegan brown sugar

- 1 teaspoon of extra virgin olive oil

For the filling:
- 2/3 tablespoons of homemade Nutella (see basic recipe)

DIRECTIONS

1. Start preparing crepes dough.

2. In a bowl pour the wholemeal flour and vegan brown sugar, mix with a spoon to mix the dry ingredients.

3. At this point, add the soymilk and with the help of a whisk, mix everything until the mixture is liquid and uniform.

4. Depending on the wholemeal flour used - which can absorb more or less liquids - you may have to add a little more milk.

5. Now, cook crepes.

6. Grease a non-stick pan with a veil of oil, eliminating any excess with a paper towel.

7. Put it on the fire, let it heat well for 1 minute: now you can pour a ladle of mixture in the centre.

8. For a pan with a diameter of 20 cm, it will be the right amount to get your crepe not too thick.

9. Let it cook for about a minute on each side, then remove it from the heat and place it on a cutting board: continue with the process until the dough is finished, placing the crepes on top of each other so that they keep well moist.

10. Fill your crepes with homemade Nutella and serve.

Cocoa crepes

PREPARATION TIME: 15 minutes
COOKING TIME: 10 minutes
CALORIES: 210

NGREDIENTS FOR 2/3 SERVINGS

- 120 gram of wholemeal flour
- 20 grams of sugar free cocoa powder
- 300 ml of soymilk
- 40 grams of wholemeal vegan brown sugar
- 1 teaspoon of extra virgin olive oil

DIRECTIONS

1. Start preparing crepes dough.
2. In a bowl, pour the wholemeal flour, cocoa powder, and vegan brown sugar, mix with a spoon to mix the dry ingredients.
3. At this point, add the soymilk and with the help of a whisk, mix everything until the mixture is liquid and uniform.
4. Depending on the wholemeal flour used - which can absorb more or less liquids - you may have to add a little more milk.
5. Now, cook crepes.
6. Grease a non-stick pan with a veil of oil, eliminating any excess with a paper towel.
7. Put it on the fire, let it heat well for 1 minute: now you can pour a ladle of mixture in the centre.
8. For a pan with a diameter of 20 cm, it will be the right amount to get your crepe not too thick.

9. Let it cook for about a minute on each side, then remove it from the heat and place it on a cutting board: continue with the process until the dough is finished, placing the crepes on top of each other so that they keep well moist.

10. Serve your crepes still hot.

Nutella and pistacchio cream cocoa crepes

PREPARATION TIME: 15 minutes
COOKING TIME: 10 minutes
CALORIES: 340

NGREDIENTS FOR 2/3 SERVINGS

- 120 gram of wholemeal flour
- 20 grams of sugar free cocoa powder
- 300 ml of soymilk
- 40 grams of wholemeal vegan brown sugar
- 1 teaspoon of extra virgin olive oil

For the filling:
- 2/3 tablespoons of homemade Nutella (see basic recipe)
- 2/3 teaspoons of homemade pistachio cream (see basic recipe)

DIRECTIONS

1. Start preparing crepes dough.
2. In a bowl, pour the wholemeal flour, cocoa powder, and vegan brown sugar, mix with a spoon to mix the dry ingredients.
3. At this point, add the soymilk and with the help of a whisk, mix everything until the mixture is liquid and uniform.
4. Depending on the wholemeal flour used - which can absorb more or less liquids - you may have to add a little more milk.
5. Now, cook crepes.
6. Grease a non-stick pan with a veil of oil, eliminating any excess with a paper towel.

7. Put it on the fire, let it heat well for 1 minute: now you can pour a ladle of mixture in the centre.

8. For a pan with a diameter of 20 cm, it will be the right amount to get your crepe not too thick.

9. Let it cook for about a minute on each side, then remove it from the heat and place it on a cutting board: continue with the process until the dough is finished, placing the crepes on top of each other so that they keep well moist.

10. Fill your crepes with 1 tablespoon of Nutella and 1 teaspoon of pistachio cream.

11. Serve your crepes still hot.

Cocoa and coconut crepes

PREPARATION TIME: 15 minutes
COOKING TIME: 10 minutes
CALORIES: 225

NGREDIENTS FOR 2/3 SERVINGS

- 100 gram of wholemeal flour
- 20 grams of coconut flour
- 20 grams of sugar free cocoa powder
- 1 pinch of vanilla powder
- 300 ml of coconut milk
- 40 grams of wholemeal vegan brown sugar
- 1 teaspoon of extra virgin olive oil
- Coconut flour (to serve)

DIRECTIONS

1. Start preparing crepes dough.
2. In a bowl pour the wholemeal flour, coconut flour, cocoa powder, vanilla powder and vegan brown sugar, mix with a spoon to mix the dry ingredients.
3. At this point, add the coconut milk and with the help of a whisk, mix everything until the mixture is liquid and uniform.
4. Depending on the wholemeal flour used - which can absorb more or less liquids - you may have to add a little more milk.
5. Now, cook crepes.

6. Grease a non-stick pan with a veil of oil, eliminating any excess with a paper towel.

7. Put it on the fire, let it heat well for 1 minute: now you can pour a ladle of mixture in the centre.

8. For a pan with a diameter of 20 cm, it will be the right amount to get your crepe not too thick.

9. Let it cook for about a minute on each side, then remove it from the heat and place it on a cutting board: continue with the process until the dough is finished, placing the crepes on top of each other so that they keep well moist.

10. Serve your crepes still hot with a sparkling of coconut flour over.

Oat and cocoa crepes

PREPARATION TIME: 15 minutes
COOKING TIME: 10 minutes
CALORIES: 210

NGREDIENTS FOR 2/3 SERVINGS

- 100 gram of oat flour
- 40 grams of sugar free cocoa powder
- 300 ml of oat milk
- 40 grams of wholemeal vegan brown sugar
- 1 teaspoon of extra virgin olive oil

DIRECTIONS

1. Start preparing crepes dough.
2. In a bowl, pour the oat flour, cocoa powder, and vegan brown sugar, mix with a spoon to mix the dry ingredients.
3. At this point, add the oat milk and with the help of a whisk, mix everything until the mixture is liquid and uniform.
4. Now, cook crepes.
5. Grease a non-stick pan with a veil of oil, eliminating any excess with a paper towel.
6. Put it on the fire, let it heat well for 1 minute: now you can pour a ladle of mixture in the centre.
7. For a pan with a diameter of 20 cm, it will be the right amount to get your crepe not too thick.

8. Let it cook for about a minute on each side, then remove it from the heat and place it on a cutting board: continue with the process until the dough is finished, placing the crepes on top of each other so that they keep well moist.

9. Serve your crepes still hot.

Almond milk chocolate and cinnamon custard

PREPARATION TIME: 10 minutes
COOKING TIME: 10 minutes
CALORIES: 250

NGREDIENTS FOR 5/6 SERVINGS

- 500 ml of almond milk
- 45 grams of corn starch
- 110 grams of vegan dark chocolate
- 3 tablespoons of brown rice syrup
- ½ teaspoon of cinnamon
- 1 pinch of salt (optional)

DIRECTIONS

1. Coarsely chop the dark chocolate with a knife.
2. Pour the corn starch, cinnamon and a pinch of salt into a saucepan.
3. Add a few tablespoons of almond milk, the minimum amount sufficient to completely dissolve the corn starch: this step will avoid the formation of lumps in the cream.
4. Pour in the remaining milk and add the chocolate.
5. Put the saucepan on the stove over low heat and cook the cream, always keeping it turned with a wooden spoon to prevent the bottom from sticking.
6. Once thickened, let it cook for another two minutes.

7. Taste the cream at this point: if you no longer feel the taste of raw starch, then remove it from the heat; otherwise continue cooking for 1 or 2 minutes.

8. Complete the cream with the rice syrup and mix well to make it incorporate.

9. Let the cream cool

10. Transfer the cream to a bowl.

11. Once your cream has cooled, it will be ready for use.

12. If it is too thick, you can mix it with a spoon or a whisk to make it nice and smooth again.

13. You can use this cream to fill your desserts or even to accompany your favorite desserts.

Chocolate and coconut custard

PREPARATION TIME: 10 minutes
COOKING TIME: 10 minutes
CALORIES: 250

NGREDIENTS FOR 5/6 SERVINGS

- 500 ml of coconut milk
- 45 grams of corn starch
- 10 grams of coconut flour
- 110 grams of vegan dark chocolate
- 3 tablespoons of brown rice syrup
- ½ teaspoon of vanilla powder

DIRECTIONS

1. Coarsely chop the dark chocolate with a knife.
2. Pour the corn starch, coconut flour, and vanilla into a saucepan.
3. Add a few tablespoons of coconut milk, the minimum amount sufficient to completely dissolve the corn starch: this step will avoid the formation of lumps in the cream.
4. Pour in the remaining milk and add the chocolate.
5. Put the saucepan on the stove over low heat and cook the cream, always keeping it turned with a wooden spoon to prevent the bottom from sticking.
6. Once thickened, let it cook for another two minutes.

7. Taste the cream at this point: if you no longer feel the taste of raw starch, then remove it from the heat; otherwise continue cooking for 1 or 2 minutes.

8. Complete the cream with the rice syrup and mix well to make it incorporate.

9. Let the cream cool.

10. Transfer the cream to a bowl.

11. Once your cream has cooled, it will be ready for use.

12. If it is too thick, you can mix it with a spoon or a whisk to make it nice and smooth again.

13. You can use this cream to fill your desserts or even to accompany your favorite desserts.

Almond and coconut pudding

PREPARATION TIME: 5 minutes
COOKING TIME: 5 minutes
CALORIES: 240

INGREDIENTS FOR 2 SERVINGS

- 80 grams of almond flour
- 1 teaspoon of coconut flour
- 1 teaspoon of coconut oil
- 40 ml of water
- 10 ml of coconut milk
- 15 grams of soy yogurt
- 5 ml of honey

DIRECTIONS

1. Fist, combine soy yogurt with almond flour, coconut oil water, coconut milk in a microwave-safe bowl.
2. Microwave for 45 seconds.
3. Then add coconut flour, honey, and microwave another 30 seconds.
4. Add additional coconut milk if necessary.
5. Serve pudding.

Flaxseed and coconut pudding

PREPARATION TIME: 5 minutes
COOKING TIME: 5 minutes
CALORIES: 220

INGREDIENTS FOR 2 SERVINGS

- 80 grams flaxseed powder

- 1 teaspoon of coconut flour

- 40 ml of water

- 10 ml of coconut milk

- 15 grams of soy yogurt

- 5 ml of honey

DIRECTIONS

1. Fist, combine soy yogurt with flax seed powder, water, coconut milk in a microwave-safe bowl.

2. Microwave for 45 seconds.

3. Then add coconut flour, honey, and microwave another 30 seconds.

4. Add additional coconut milk if necessary.

5. Serve pudding.

Flaxseed and almond pudding

PREPARATION TIME: 5 minutes
COOKING TIME: 5 minutes
CALORIES: 280

INGREDIENTS FOR 2 SERVINGS

- 60 grams flaxseed powder
- 25 grams of almond flour
- 40 ml of water
- 10 ml of almond milk
- 15 grams of soy yogurt
- 5 ml of honey
- 20 grams of sliced almond (to serve)

DIRECTIONS

1. Fist, combine soy yogurt with flax seed powder, water, almond milk in a microwave-safe bowl.
2. Microwave for 45 seconds.
3. Then add almond flour, honey, and microwave another 30 seconds.
4. Add additional almond milk if necessary.
5. Serve pudding with a topping of sliced almonds.

Flaxseed and chocolate pudding

PREPARATION TIME: 10 minutes
COOKING TIME: 5 minutes
CALORIES: 240

INGREDIENTS FOR 2 SERVINGS

- 60 grams of flaxseed powder

- 50 ml water

- 10 grams of coconut flour

- 10 grams of sugar free cocoa

- 10 ml of soymilk

- 15 grams of soy yogurt

- 5 ml of honey

- 10 grams of vegan chocolate chips

- 100 grams of berries

DIRECTIONS

1. Fist, put soy yogurt in a microwave-safe bowl

2. Then, add flax seed powder, water, soymilk and cocoa powder.

3. Microwave for 45 seconds.

4. Then add coconut flour, honey, and microwave another 30 seconds.

5. Add additional soymilk if necessary.

6. Meanwhile, clean berries.

7. When it is ready, serve pudding with vegan chocolate chips and berries.

Chocolate and coconut pudding

PREPARATION TIME: 5 minutes
COOKING TIME: 8 minutes
REST TIME: 2 hours
CALORIES: 200

INGREDIENTS FOR 2 SERVINGS

- 35 grams of sugar free cocoa powder
- 35 grams of corn starch
- 60 grams of coconut sugar
- 1 pinch salt
- 250 ml of coconut milk
- 60 grams of vegan chocolate chips
- 1/2 tablespoon of vanilla extract

DIRECTIONS

1. First, in a medium saucepan with the heat off, thoroughly whisk together cocoa powder, coconut sugar, corn starch, and salt, working to remove all lumps.
2. Gradually pour in the coconut milk in small amounts, whisking after each addition until it is smooth.
3. Turn the heat to medium and bring to a simmer, stirring frequently.
4. Once it just starts to bubble on the edges, reduce the heat to low.
5. Cook; stirring often, until thickened, about 2 minutes (make sure to stir into the edges of the pan so it does not stick).

6. The pudding will continue to thicken and set as it cools, so it does not need to be fully thick at this point.
7. Remove from the heat and stir in the chocolate chips and vanilla, stirring until fully melted.
8. Transfer to a container and press plastic wrap or wax paper on the surface (this prevents a film from forming on the top).
9. Refrigerate 2 hours until cold and set.

Dark chocolate pudding

PREPARATION TIME: 10 minutes
COOKING TIME: 20 minutes
CALORIES: 270

INGREDIENTS FOR 2 SERVINGS

- 500 ml almond milk
- 65 grams vegan brown sugar
- 50 grams of vegan dark chocolate
- 25 grams of sugar free cocoa
- 15 grams of potato starch
- 1 cup of coffee (or ½ teaspoon of instant coffee)
- ½ teaspoon of agar agar
- 1 pinch of vanilla powder

DIRECTIONS

1. In a saucepan, pour the potato starch, cocoa, agar agar, vanilla and add a little almond milk enough to dissolve all the powders well, mixing well with a wooden or silicone spoon.
2. Then gradually add the rest of the almond milk, taking care to eliminate any lumps.
3. Add the brown sugar, coffee and coarsely chopped dark chocolate.
4. Put the saucepan over medium heat and continue stirring until the cream has thickened and reached a boil.

5. At that point, continue cooking for another 2 minutes, turn off the heat and pour the mixture into the pudding molds.
6. Let them cool at room temperature for an hour and then put them in the refrigerator for at least a couple of hours.
7. Turn out the puddings on a saucer and serve.

Pistachio and chocolate pudding

PREPARATION TIME: 10 minutes
COOKING TIME: 20 minutes
CALORIES: 290

INGREDIENTS FOR 2 SERVINGS

- 500 ml of coconut milk
- 65 grams vegan brown sugar
- 50 grams of vegan dark chocolate
- 25 grams of sugar free cocoa
- 15 grams of potato starch
- 30 grams of chopped pistachios
- ½ teaspoon of agar agar
- 1 pinch of vanilla powder

DIRECTIONS

1. In a saucepan, pour the potato starch, cocoa, agar agar, vanilla and add a little coconut milk enough to dissolve all the powders well, mixing well with a wooden or silicone spoon.
2. Then gradually add the rest of the coconut milk, taking care to eliminate any lumps.
3. Add the brown sugar, chopped pistachios and coarsely chopped dark chocolate.
4. Put the saucepan over medium heat and continue stirring until the cream has thickened and reached a boil.

5. At that point, continue cooking for another 2 minutes, turn off the heat and pour the mixture into the pudding molds.
6. Let them cool at room temperature for an hour and then put them in the refrigerator for at least a couple of hours.
7. Turn out the puddings on a saucer and serve.

Corn starch and cocoa pudding

PREPARATION TIME: 5 minutes
COOKING TIME: 8 minutes
REST TIME: 2 hours
CALORIES:200

INGREDIENTS FOR 2 SERVINGS

- 35 grams of sugar free cocoa powder
- 35 grams of corn starch
- 60 grams of vegan brown sugar
- 1 pinch salt
- 250 ml of homemade corn milk (see basic recipe)
- 60 grams of vegan chocolate chips
- 1/2 tablespoon of vanilla extract

DIRECTIONS

1. First, in a medium saucepan with the heat off, thoroughly whisk together cocoa powder, brown sugar, corn starch, and salt, working to remove all lumps.
2. Gradually pour in the corn milk in small amounts, whisking after each addition until it is smooth.
3. Turn the heat to medium and bring to a simmer, stirring frequently.
4. Once it just starts to bubble on the edges, reduce the heat to low.
5. Cook; stirring often, until thickened, about 2 minutes (make sure to stir into the edges of the pan so it does not stick).

6. The pudding will continue to thicken and set as it cools, so it does not need to be fully thick at this point.

7. Remove from the heat and stir in the chocolate chips and vanilla, stirring until fully melted.

8. Transfer to a container and press plastic wrap or wax paper on the surface (this prevents a film from forming on the top).

9. Refrigerate 2 hours until cold and set.

Nuts and berries oatmeal

PREPARATION TIME: 10 minutes
COOKING TIME: 20 minutes
CALORIES: 270

INGREDIENTS FOR 2 SERVINGS

- 50 grams of mixed nuts (almonds, hazelnuts and pistachios)
- 60 grams of whole oat flakes
- 20 grams of flaxseed powder
- 10 ml of agave syrup
- 10 grams of pumpkin seeds
- 40 grams of berries

DIRECTIONS

1. First, finely chop the dried fruit, then the almonds, hazelnuts and pistachios.
2. You can also decide to use just one type of dried fruit to prepare your recipe.
3. In a bowl, pour the whole oat flakes, flaxseed powder, and the freshly chopped dried fruit.
4. Add the pumpkin seeds.
5. Wash berries than cut into pieces
6. Now, add berries in the mixture.
7. Mix everything with the agave syrup.
8. Min until you will have a soft and sticky mixture.

9. Roll out the mixture just obtained on a baking tray covered with baking paper with the help of slightly moistened hands or with the back of a spoon always wet, and bake (static oven) at 180 ° C for about 20 minutes, at the end leave cool and put it in a jar breaking it into irregular blocks.

10. You can serve your oatmeal with a plant-based yogurt or milk.

Pistachios and raspberries oatmeal

PREPARATION TIME: 10 minutes
COOKING TIME: 20 minutes
CALORIES: 285

INGREDIENTS FOR 2 SERVINGS

- 50 grams of chopped pistachios
- 60 grams of whole oat flakes
- 20 grams of flaxseed powder
- 1 teaspoon of marble syrup
- 10 grams of pumpkin seeds
- 60 grams of raspberries

DIRECTIONS

1. First, finely chop pistachios.
2. In a bowl, pour the whole oat flakes, flaxseed powder, and the freshly chopped pistachios.
3. Add the pumpkin seeds.
4. Wash raspberries than cut into pieces
5. Now, add raspberries in the mixture.
6. Mix everything with the marble syrup.
7. Min until you will have a soft and sticky mixture.
8. Roll out the mixture just obtained on a baking tray covered with baking paper with the help of slightly moistened hands or with the back of a spoon always wet, and bake (static oven) at 180 ° C for about 20

minutes, at the end leave cool and put it in a jar breaking it into irregular blocks.

9. You can serve your oatmeal with a plant-based yogurt or milk.

Berries and apples oatmeal

PREPARATION TIME: 15 minutes
COOKING TIME: 40 minutes
CALORIES: 250

INGREDIENTS FOR 4 SERVINGS

- 50 grams of oat flour
- 30 grams of rolled oats
- 70 grams of vegan brown sugar
- 1 pinch of salt
- 30 grams of sun flower oil
- 300 grams of frozen whole mixed berries
- 16 slice of apple
- 20 ml of fresh lemon juice
- 25 grams of corn starch

DIRECTIONS

1. Start the recipe combining the oat flour, rolled oats, 50 grams of brown sugar, and salt in a bowl and stir.
2. Use a pastry blender or fork to work the butter into the flour until the crust reaches a uniform crumbly consistency to make the topping.
3. Transfer the bowl to the freezer.
4. Toss the frozen berries and apples with the remaining 20 grams of brown sugar, lemon juice, and corn starch in a separate bowl.
5. Pour this mixture into a 1 1/2-qt. casserole dish.

6. Bake at 185° C for 30 minutes.

7. When the cooking time is complete, top the fruit with the topping from the freezer.

8. Take all ingredients into a baking pan.

9. Heat up oven temperature to 200° C.

10. Let cook for at least 10 minutes.

11. Let the crisp cool before serving.

Vanilla and apples oatmeal

PREPARATION TIME: 15 minutes
COOKING TIME: 40 minutes
CALORIES: 250

INGREDIENTS FOR 4 SERVINGS

- 50 grams of oat flour
- 30 grams of rolled oats
- 70 grams of vegan brown sugar
- 1 pinch of salt
- 30 grams of sun flower oil
- 16 slice of apple
- 1 teaspoon of vanilla powder
- 20 ml of fresh lemon juice
- 25 grams of corn starch

DIRECTIONS

1. Start the recipe combining the oat flour, rolled oats, 50 grams of brown sugar, and salt in a bowl and stir.
2. Use a pastry blender or fork to work the butter into the flour until the crust reaches a uniform crumbly consistency to make the topping.
3. Transfer the bowl to the freezer.
4. Toss the apples with the remaining 20 grams of brown sugar, lemon juice, vanilla powder, and corn starch in a separate bowl.
5. Pour this mixture into a 1 1/2-qt. casserole dish.

6. Bake at 185° C for 30 minutes.

7. When the cooking time is complete, top the fruit with the topping from the freezer.

8. Take all ingredients into a baking pan.

9. Heat up oven temperature to 200° C.

10. Let cook for at least 10 minutes.

11. Let the crisp cool before serving.

Strawberry and apricot porridge

PREPARATION TIME: 10 minutes
REST TIME: one night
CALORIES: 280

INGREDIENTS FOR 2 SERVINGS

- 160 grams of oat flakes
- 480 grams of soy yogurt
- 200 grams of vegetable soymilk
- 100 grams of strawberries
- ½ apple
- 4 apricots
- 40 grams of almonds
- Maple syrup to taste

DIRECTIONS

1. If you want to taste the porridge recipe, you have to start preparing it the previous evening.
2. Mix the oat flakes in a bowl with the soy yogurt and soymilk, cover with plastic wrap and place in the refrigerator to rest overnight.
3. In the morning, wash and peel the fruit. Remove any waste parts and cut the fruit into cubes.
4. Distribute the porridge in 4 bowls and complete each with a little maple syrup (or another sweetener to taste), strawberries, apple and apricots, spreading all over the surface of the porridge.
5. You can serve

Berries and pear porridge

PREPARATION TIME: 10 minutes
REST TIME: one night
CALORIES: 280

INGREDIENTS FOR 2 SERVINGS

- 160 grams of oat flakes
- 480 grams of soy yogurt
- 200 grams of vegetable soymilk
- 100 grams of mixed berries
- 2 pears
- 40 grams of walnuts
- Maple syrup to taste

DIRECTIONS

1. If you want to taste the porridge recipe, you have to start preparing it the previous evening.
2. Mix the oat flakes in a bowl with the soy yogurt and soymilk, cover with plastic wrap and place in the refrigerator to rest overnight.
3. In the morning, wash and peel the fruit. Remove any waste parts and cut the fruit into cubes.
4. Distribute the porridge in 4 bowls and complete each with a little maple syrup (or another sweetener to taste), berries and pears pieces, spreading all over the surface of the porridge.
5. You can serve your porridge.

Peanut butter and quinoa porridge

PREPARATION TIME: 10 minutes
COOKING TIME: 10 minutes
CALORIES: 280

INGREDIENTS FOR 2 SERVINGS

- 40 grams of de-oiled soy flakes
- 50 grams of wholemeal barley flakes
- 15 grams of carob flour
- 10 grams of flaxseed powder
- 2 bananas
- 1 pinch of cinnamon
- 100 ml of water
- 120 ml of rice milk
- 20 grams of all natural homemade peanut butter (see basic recipe)
- puffed quinoa

DIRECTIONS

1. Put the soy flakes and whole barley flakes in a saucepan.
2. Add the carob flour, cinnamon powder, flaxseed powder and 1 banana mashed well with a fork.
3. Pour in the water and 100 ml of rice milk and mix.
4. Turn on the heat and cook until the mixture has thickened and the flakes are soft.

5. Transfer the porridge to a bowl, completing with the rice milk (20 ml), the remaining banana cut into slices, the peanut butter and a handful of puffed quinoa.
6. Serve immediately.

Peanut butter and cocoa porridge

PREPARATION TIME: 10 minutes
COOKING TIME: 10 minutes
CALORIES: 280

INGREDIENTS FOR 2 SERVINGS

- 40 grams of de-oiled soy flakes
- 50 grams of wholemeal barley flakes
- 15 grams of carob flour
- 10 grams of flaxseed powder
- 1 tablespoon of sugar free cocoa powder
- 1 pinch of vanilla powder
- 100 grams of soy yogurt
- 100 ml of water
- 120 ml of soymilk
- 20 grams of homemade peanut butter (see basic recipe)

DIRECTIONS

1. Put the soy flakes and whole barley flakes in a saucepan.
2. Add the carob flour, vanilla powder, cocoa, flaxseed powder and half of soy yogurt with a fork.
3. Pour in the water and 100 ml of soymilk and mix.
4. Turn on the heat and cook until the mixture has thickened and the flakes are soft.

5. Transfer the porridge to a bowl, completing with the rice milk (20 ml), the remaining soy yogurt and the peanut butter.

6. Serve immediately.

Lime and apple cream

PREPARATION TIME: 10 minutes
COOKING TIME: 10 minutes
CALORIES: 190
INGREDIENTS FOR 4 SERVINGS

- 4 apples
- the juice of two limes
- the grated zest of a lime
- 12 hazelnuts
- 1 tablespoon of sugar free cocoa powder
- orange slices (for garnish)

DIRECTIONS

1. Peel the apples and cut them into large chunks.
2. Separately, after grating the peel of one of the two limes, squeeze them and keep the juice aside.
3. Place a non-stick pan on medium heat and cook the apples together with the lime juice and add the grated zest.
4. Let the fruit cook until it becomes soft but not pulped.
5. Chop the hazelnuts with a knife or with a mixer equipped with blades.
6. With an immersion blender, mix the apples until they are reduced to a cream and place them in small bowls.
7. Decorate the cream with chopped hazelnuts and a generous sprinkling of bitter cocoa.
8. If you want, you can decorate the portions with small slices of orange or with zest of the same.

Orange and apple cream

PREPARATION TIME: 10 minutes
COOKING TIME: 10 minutes
CALORIES: 190

INGREDIENTS FOR 4 SERVINGS

- 4 apples
- the juice of two oranges
- the grated zest of a orange
- 1 pinch of cinnamon
- 12 almonds
- orange slices (for garnish)

DIRECTIONS

1. Peel the apples and cut them into large chunks.
2. Separately, after grating the peel of one of the two oranges, squeeze them and keep the juice aside.
3. Place a non-stick pan on medium heat, cook the apples together with the cinnamon, orange juice, and add the grated zest.
4. Let the fruit cook until it becomes soft but not pulped.
5. Chop the almonds with a knife or with a mixer equipped with blades.
6. With an immersion blender, mix the apples until they are reduced to a cream and place them in small bowls.
7. Decorate the cream with chopped almonds.
8. If you want, you can decorate the portions with small slices of orange or with zest of the same.

Avocado and cucumber cream

PREPARATION TIME: 15 minutes+ 60 minutes rest in the fridge
CALORIES: 310

INGREDIENTS FOR 2 SERVINGS

- 1 avocado
- 1 cucumber
- Juice of one orange
- 100 ml of soymilk
- 1 tsp salt
- 2 tsp chia seeds
- 200 ml of cold vegetable broth

DIRECTIONS

1. First, halve the avocado, pit it and remove the pulp from the peel.
2. Peel and cut the cucumber into slices.
3. Squeeze orange juice as well.
4. Transfer all the ingredients (avocado, cucumber, orange juice, soymilk, vegetable broth, salt) with stems included, and broth in a measuring container.
5. Leave to rest in the fridge for about 60 minutes.
6. After this time, take the ingredients and blend them with an immersion blender.
7. Blend all ingredients until obtain a thick cream.
8. When it is done you can serve.

Almond and cocoa hummus

PREPARATION TIME: 10 minutes
REST TIME: 5 minutes
CALORIES: 290

INGREDIENTS FOR 5 SERVINGS

- 225 grams of boiled chickpeas
- 120 ml of agave syrup
- 20 grams of sugar free cocoa powder
- 3 tablespoons of water
- 2 tablespoons of all natural homemade almond cream (see basic recipe)
- 1 sprinkle of cinnamon
- 1 pinch of vanilla powder
- 1 pinch of salt
- Chopped almonds (to decorate)

DIRECTIONS

1. If you do not have them ready, boil the chickpeas before starting the recipe.
2. When they will be ready let, them cool.
3. Pour the chickpeas, agave syrup, cocoa, water, almond cream, cinnamon, vanilla and salt into the kitchen mixer.
4. Run the mixer and blend the mixture for a few minutes until you get a smooth and homogeneous cream.

5. If necessary, you can adjust the final flavour of your hummus by adding more cocoa or syrup or almond cream depending on your taste.

6. Alternatively, add more water if you prefer the softer cream. In the meantime, peel and finely chop the almonds (and a couple of tablespoons will suffice).

7. Transfer the chocolate and almond hummus to a bowl and decorate the surface with chopped almonds

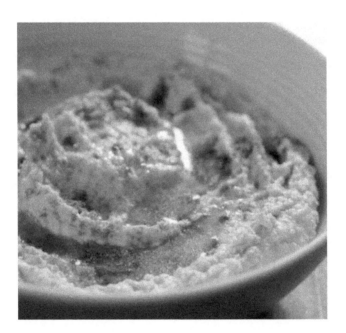

Pistachio and cocoa hummus

PREPARATION TIME: 10 minutes
REST TIME: 5 minutes
CALORIES: 290

INGREDIENTS FOR 5 SERVINGS

- 225 grams of boiled chickpeas
- 120 ml of agave syrup
- 20 grams of sugar free cocoa powder
- 3 tablespoons of water
- 2 tablespoons of all natural pistachio cream (see basic) recipe
- 1 pinch of vanilla powder
- 1 pinch of salt
- Chopped almonds (to decorate)

DIRECTIONS

1. If you do not have them ready, boil the chickpeas before starting the recipe.
2. When they will be ready let, them cool.
3. Pour the chickpeas, agave syrup, cocoa, water, pistachio cream, vanilla and salt into the kitchen mixer.
4. Run the mixer and blend the mixture for a few minutes until you get a smooth and homogeneous cream.
5. If necessary, you can adjust the final flavour of your hummus by adding more cocoa or syrup or almond cream depending on your taste.

6. Or add more water if you prefer the softer cream. In the meantime, peel and finely chop the almonds (and a couple of tablespoons will suffice).
7. Transfer the chocolate and almond hummus to a bowl and decorate the surface with chopped almonds

Hummus and coffee cream

PREPARATION TIME: 10 minutes
REST TIME: 60 minutes
CALORIES: 260

INGREDIENTS FOR 4 SERVINGS

- 200 grams of boiled chickpeas without salt
- 1 cup of coffee
- 2 tablespoons of brown rice syrup
- 2 tablespoons of all natural hazelnut cream (see basic recipe)
- 1 teaspoon of instant coffee
- ¼ teaspoon of vanilla powder

DIRECTIONS

1. If you do not have them ready, boil the chickpeas in boiling water, then drain them.
2. Let them cool and transfer them to the food processor.
3. Always in the food processor, combine all the ingredients: chickpeas, coffee, instant coffee, hazelnut cream, rice syrup and vanilla.
4. Operate the food processor and blend until you get a soft and perfectly smooth cream.
5. Transfer the hummus into a bowl and place it in the refrigerator to rest for at least an hour. If you like, decorate with coffee beans and serve.

Hummus and Nutella cream

PREPARATION TIME: 10 minutes
REST TIME: 60 minutes
CALORIES: 320

INGREDIENTS FOR 4 SERVINGS

- 200 grams of boiled chickpeas without salt

- 1 cup of almond flour

- 2 tablespoons of brown rice syrup

- 2 tablespoons of homemade Nutella cream (see basic recipe)

- 1 teaspoon of vanilla powder

- 20 grams of vegan dark chocolate chips (optional)

DIRECTIONS

1. If you do not have them ready, boil the chickpeas in boiling water, and then drain them.
2. Let them cool and transfer them to the food processor.
3. Always in the food processor, combine all the ingredients: chickpeas, almond flour, vanilla powder, and Nutella cream and rice syrup.
4. Operate the food processor and blend until you get a soft and perfectly smooth cream.
5. Transfer the hummus into a bowl and place it in the refrigerator to rest for at least an hour.
6. If you like, decorate with dark chocolate chips and serve.

Almond milk and strawberry scones

PREPARATION TIME: 25 minutes
COOKING TIME: 30 minutes
CALORIES: 430

INGREDIENTS FOR 6 SERVINGS

- 250 grams of whole meal flour
- 30 grams of vegan brown sugar
- 6 grams of natural Baking Powder
- 1 pinch of salt
- 70 grams of sunflower oil
- 70 ml of almond milk
- 200 grams of soymilk whipped cream
- 250 grams of strawberries homemade jam (see recipe)

DIRECTIONS

1. First, sift together the wholemeal flour, brown sugar, baking powder, and salt, in a medium-size bowl.
2. Add the sunflower oil and combine with a fork.
3. Use a fork, your fingers, or a pastry blender to work the butter into the flour until the mixture resembles coarse crumbs.
4. Add the almond milk and stir with a fork until the ingredients are just moistened.
5. Gather the dough together and press it gently into a rough ball.
6. Turn the dough out onto a lightly floured surface, flour your hands, and pat the dough together.

7. The dough may still be crumbly.

8. Knead the dough gently until it just comes together and then shape it into a rectangle shape.

9. Use a lightly floured rolling pin to roll the dough to a thickness of about ¾ in.

10. Cut the dough crosswise into three portions and then cut each portion into two triangle shapes.

11. You should have six generously sized scones.

12. Put the scones in a baking pan and let cook at 190° C. for 25 minutes (at least).

13. Check the cooking and if they are not ready, keep for other 5 minutes.

14. Meanwhile, whip the soymilk whipped cream from the fridge.

15. When scones will be done, let them cool.

16. Then halve the scones and spread the jam in the half.

17. Add the whipped cream and close scones with the other half.

18. You can serve them

Coconut scones with hazelnut cream

PREPARATION TIME: 25 minutes
COOKING TIME: 30 minutes
CALORIES: 540

INGREDIENTS FOR 6 SERVINGS

- 200 grams of whole meal flour

- 50 grams of coconut flour

- 30 grams of vegan brown sugar

- 6 grams of natural Baking Powder

- 1 pinch of salt

- 70 grams of sunflower oil

- 70 ml of coconut milk

- 200 grams of soymilk whipped cream

- 120 grams of homemade hazelnut cream (see basic recipe)

DIRECTIONS

1. First, sift together the wholemeal flour, coconut flour, brown sugar, baking powder, and salt, in a medium-size bowl.

2. Add the sunflower oil and combine with a fork.

3. Use a fork, your fingers, or a pastry blender to work the butter into the flour until the mixture resembles coarse crumbs.

4. Add the coconut milk and stir with a fork until the ingredients are just moistened.

5. Gather the dough together and press it gently into a rough ball.

6. Turn the dough out onto a lightly floured surface, flour your hands, and pat the dough together.

7. The dough may still be crumbly.

8. Knead the dough gently until it just comes together and then shape it into a rectangle shape.

9. Use a lightly floured rolling pin to roll the dough to a thickness of about ¾ in.

10. Cut the dough crosswise into three portions and then cut each portion into two triangle shapes.

11. You should have six generously sized scones.

12. Put the scones in a baking pan and let cook at 190° C. for 25 minutes (at least).

13. Check the cooking and if they are not ready, keep for other 5 minutes.

14. Meanwhile, whip the soymilk whipped cream from the fridge.

15. When scones will be done, let them cool.

16. Then halve the scones and spread the hazelnut cream in the half.

17. Add the whipped cream and close scones with the other half.

18. You can serve them.

Soy and chocolate scones

PREPARATION TIME: 25 minutes
COOKING TIME: 30 minutes
CALORIES: 490

INGREDIENTS FOR 6 SERVINGS

- 200 grams of whole meal flour
- 50 grams of soy flour
- 30 grams of vegan brown sugar
- 6 grams of natural Baking Powder
- 1 pinch of salt
- 70 grams of sunflower oil
- 70 ml of soymilk
- 200 grams of soymilk whipped cream
- 50 grams of vegan chocolate chips

DIRECTIONS

1. First, sift together the wholemeal flour, soy flour, brown sugar, baking powder, and salt, in a medium-size bowl.
2. Add the sunflower oil and combine with a fork.
3. Use a fork, your fingers, or a pastry blender to work the butter into the flour until the mixture resembles coarse crumbs.
4. Add the soymilk and stir with a fork until the ingredients are just moistened.
5. Gather the dough together and press it gently into a rough ball.

6. Turn the dough out onto a lightly floured surface, flour your hands, and pat the dough together.

7. The dough may still be crumbly.

8. Knead the dough gently until it just comes together and then shape it into a rectangle shape.

9. Use a lightly floured rolling pin to roll the dough to a thickness of about ¾ in.

10. Cut the dough crosswise into three portions and then cut each portion into two triangle shapes.

11. You should have six generously sized scones.

12. Put the scones in a baking pan and let cook at 190° C. for 25 minutes (at least).

13. Check the cooking and if they are not ready, keep for other 5 minutes.

14. Meanwhile, whip the soymilk whipped cream from the fridge.

15. Melt soymilk whipped cream with vegan chocolate chips.

16. When scones will be done, let them cool.

17. Then halve the scones and spread with the chocolate chips whipped cream and close scones with the other half.

18. You can serve them.

Almonds muffins

PREPARATION TIME: 15 minutes
COOKING TIME: 20 minutes
CALORIES: 390

INGREDIENTS FOR 4/5 SERVINGS

- 150 grams of wholemeal flour

- 75 grams of almond flour

- 80 grams of raw cane vegan sugar

- 50 grams of chopped almonds

- 200 ml of almond milk

- 50 g of sunflower oil

- ½ sachet of yeast (cream of tartar)

- a pinch of Cinnamon

- 1 pinch of salt

DIRECTIONS

1. First, prepare the dough.

2. If you do not have almond grain ready, you can prepare it by yourself, peeling the almonds and chopping them finely.

3. Toast the chopped almonds in a hot pan until golden.

4. In a bowl, combine the wholemeal flour, almond flour, brown sugar, baking powder, a pinch of cinnamon and salt.

5. Mix everything with a wooden spoon, and then add the almond milk and sunflower oil and mix.

6. Finally add the chopped almonds and incorporate it well into the dough.

7. Line the muffin molds with paper cups, fill them with the dough up to three quarters, and decorate the surface with slicedalmonds.

8. Bake in a static oven at 190 ° C for about 20 minutes.

9. Always check the cooking and if they are cooked, take the almond muffins out of the oven.

10. Let the muffins cool, and then remove them from the mold to cool completely.

11. You can serve your muffins cold.

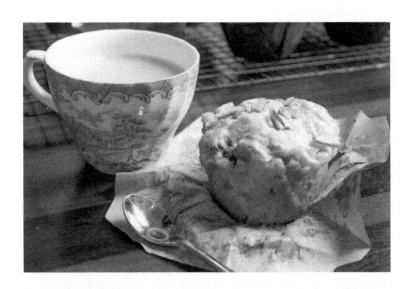

Almonds and coconut muffins

PREPARATION TIME: 15 minutes
COOKING TIME: 20 minutes
CALORIES: 410

INGREDIENTS FOR 4/5 SERVINGS

- 50 grams of wholemeal flour

- 100 grams of almond flour

- 75 grams of coconut flour

- 80 grams of raw cane vegan sugar

- 50 grams of chopped almonds

- 200 ml of coconut milk

- 50 g of sunflower oil

- ½ sachet of yeast (cream of tartar)

- a pinch of nutmeg

- 1 pinch of salt

- Coconut flour (to decorate)

DIRECTIONS

1. First, prepare muffins dough.

2. If you do not have almond grain ready, you can prepare it by yourself, peeling the almonds and chopping them finely.

3. Toast the chopped almonds in a hot pan until golden.

4. In a bowl, combine the wholemeal flour, almond flour, coconut brown sugar, baking powder, a pinch of nutmeg and salt.

5. Mix everything with a wooden spoon, and then add the coconut milk and sunflower oil and mix.

6. Finally add the chopped almonds and incorporate it well into the dough.

7. Line the muffin molds with paper cups, fill them with the dough up to three quarters, and decorate the surface with slicedalmonds.

8. Bake in a static oven at 190 ° C for about 20 minutes.

9. Always check the cooking and if they are cooked, take the almond muffins out of the oven.

10. Let the muffins cool, and then remove them from the mold to cool completely.

11. You can serve your muffins cold with a sprinkle of coconut flour over.

Almonds and chocolate muffins

PREPARATION TIME: 15 minutes
COOKING TIME: 20 minutes
CALORIES: 390

INGREDIENTS FOR 4/5 SERVINGS

- 150 grams of wholemeal flour
- 60 grams of almond flour
- 15 grams of sugar free cocoa powder
- 80 grams of raw cane vegan sugar
- 50 grams of vegan dark chocolate (chopped)
- 200 ml of almond milk
- 50 g of sunflower oil
- ½ sachet of yeast (cream of tartar)
- a pinch of vanilla powder
- 1 pinch of salt

DIRECTIONS

1. If you do not have almond grain ready, you can prepare it by yourself, peeling the almonds and chopping them finely.
2. Meanwhile, chop vegan dark chocolate too.
3. In a bowl, combine the wholemeal flour, almond flour, cocoa powder, brown sugar, baking powder, a pinch of vanilla and salt.
4. Mix everything with a wooden spoon, and then add the almond milk and sunflower oil and mix.

5. Finally add the chopped chocolate and incorporate it well into the dough.
6. Line the muffin molds with paper cups, fill them with the dough up to three quarters, and decorate the surface with slicedalmonds.
7. Bake in a static oven at 190 ° C for about 20 minutes.
8. Always check the cooking and if they are cooked, take the almond muffins out of the oven.
9. Let the muffins cool, and then remove them from the mold to cool completely.
10. You can serve your muffins cold.

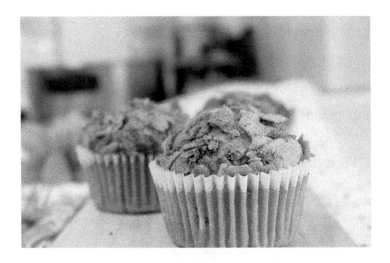

Spelt and agave syrup muffins

PREPARATION TIME: 15 minutes
COOKING TIME: 30 minutes
CALORIES: 340

INGREDIENTS FOR 4/5 SERVINGS

- 150 grams of whole wheat flour

- zest of one lemon

- 150 grams of wholemeal spelt flour

- 120 ml of agave syrup

- 1 sachet of yeast

- 1 pinch of salt

- 120 ml of sunflower oil

- spelt milk to taste

DIRECTIONS

1. Wash and take lemon zest.

2. In a large bowl, pour all the dry ingredients (whole meal flour, lemon zest, spelt flour, yeast and salt) and mix.

3. Then add the spelt milk, the oil and the agave syrup and mix again until you get a soft and homogeneous consistency.

4. Transfer the mixture into muffin mold.

5. Bake your muffins at 180 ° C for about 30 minutes in a static oven.

6. Let them cool and serve.

Spelt and pistachio muffins

PREPARATION TIME: 15 minutes
COOKING TIME: 30 minutes
CALORIES: 340

INGREDIENTS FOR 4/5 SERVINGS

- 100 grams of whole wheat flour
- zest of one lemon
- 150 grams of wholemeal spelt flour
- 50 grams of finely chopped pistachios
- 100 ml of marble syrup
- 20 ml of almond milk
- 1 sachet of yeast
- 1 pinch of salt
- 120 ml of sunflower oil
- spelt milk to taste

DIRECTIONS

1. If you don't' have chopped pistachios, you can have it by your own.
2. Peel and chop very finely 50 grams of pistachios.
3. Meanwhile wash and take lemon zest.
4. In a large bowl, pour all the dry ingredients (whole meal flour, lemon zest, spelt flour, chopped pistachios, yeast and salt) and mix.
5. Then add the spelt milk, almond milk the oil and the agave syrup and mix again until you get a soft and homogeneous consistency.
6. Transfer the mixture into muffin mold.

7. Bake your muffins at 180 ° C for about 30 minutes in a static oven.

8. Let them cool and serve.

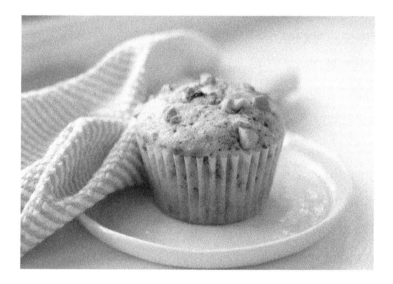

Carrot and pecans muffins

PREPARATION TIME: 15 minutes
COOKING TIME: 30/35 minutes
CALORIES: 390

INGREDIENTS FOR 4 SERVINGS

- 200 grams of wholemeal flour
- 20 grams of flaxseed powder
- 90 grams of vegan brown sugar
- 10 grams of corn starch
- 1 pinch of baking powder
- Zest of ½ organic orange
- 1 clean carrots
- 40 grams of pecans
- 50 ml orange juice
- 120 ml of soymilk (or other vegetable milk)
- 60 grams of vegetal oil
- 1 pinch of vanilla powder
- 1 pinch of salt

DIRECTIONS

1. In a bowl, combine the wholemeal flour, flaxseed powder, brown vegan sugar, corn starch, baking powder, vanilla and salt and give a first stir.
2. Now, chop very coarsely the pecans.
3. Peel, wash and grate the carrots with the wide hole grater.

4. Add pecans, carrots and orange zest to the dry ingredients and mix again.

5. Finally, add the orange juice, the soymilk and the vegetal oil and mix until everything is combined and obtain a smooth mixture.

6. Pour the muffin mixture into large cups and bake in a static oven at 190 °C for 30-35 minutes.

7. To check that they are actually cooked, do the toothpick test: stick one in the centre of a muffin and if it comes out completely dry, they will be ready.

8. If you use normal sized cups, cooking times will be shortened by a few minutes.

9. Serve muffins warm.

Carrot and almonds muffins

PREPARATION TIME: 15 minutes
COOKING TIME: 30/35 minutes
CALORIES: 410

INGREDIENTS FOR 4 SERVINGS

- 160 grams of wholemeal flour

- 60 grams of almond flour

- 90 grams of vegan brown sugar

- 10 grams of corn starch

- 1 pinch of baking powder

- Zest of ½ organic orange

- 1 clean carrots

- 40 grams of almonds

- 50 ml orange juice

- 120 ml of almond milk

- 60 grams of vegetal oil

- 1 pinch of vanilla powder

- 1 pinch of salt

DIRECTIONS

1. In a bowl, combine the wholemeal flour, almond flour, brown vegan sugar, corn starch, baking powder, vanilla and salt and give a first stir.

2. Now peel and chop very coarsely the almonds.

3. Peel, wash and grate the carrots with the wide hole grater.

4. Add pecans, carrots and orange zest to the dry ingredients and mix again.

5. Finally, add the orange juice, the almond milk and the vegetal oil and mix until everything is combined and obtain a smooth mixture.

6. Pour the muffin mixture into large cups and bake in a static oven at 190 °C for 30-35 minutes.

7. To check that they are actually cooked, do the toothpick test: stick one in the centre of a muffin and if it comes out completely dry, they will be ready.

8. If you use normal sized cups, cooking times will be shortened by a few minutes.

9. Serve muffins warm.

Orange carrot and chocolate muffins

PREPARATION TIME: 15 minutes
COOKING TIME: 30/35 minutes
CALORIES: 450

INGREDIENTS FOR 4 SERVINGS

- 200 grams of wholemeal flour
- 20 grams of sugar free cocoa powder
- 90 grams of vegan brown sugar
- 10 grams of corn starch
- 1 pinch of baking powder
- Zest of ½ organic orange
- 1 clean carrots
- 40 grams of vegan dark chocolate chips
- 50 ml orange juice
- 120 ml of rice milk
- 60 grams of vegetal oil
- 1 pinch of vanilla powder
- 1 pinch of salt

DIRECTIONS

1. In a bowl, combine the wholemeal flour, cocoa powder, brown vegan sugar, corn starch, baking powder, vanilla and salt and give a first stir.
2. Peel, wash and grate the carrots with the wide hole grater.

3. Add dark chocolate chips, carrots and orange zest to the dry ingredients and mix again.
4. Finally, add the orange juice, the rice milk and the vegetal oil and mix until everything is combined and obtain a smooth mixture.
5. Pour the muffin mixture into large cups and bake in a static oven at 190 °C for 30-35 minutes.
6. To check that they are actually cooked, do the toothpick test: stick one in the centre of a muffin and if it comes out completely dry, they will be ready.
7. If you use normal sized cups, cooking times will be shortened by a few minutes.
8. Serve muffins warm.

Pear and hazelnut muffins

PREPARATION TIME: 15 minutes
COOKING TIME: 30 minutes
CALORIES: 415

INGREDIENTS FOR 4 SERVINGS

- 300 grams of wholemeal flour
- zest of an untreated organic lemon
- 120 ml of maple syrup
- 1 sachet of cream of tartar
- 1 pinch of salt
- 120 ml of sunflower oil
- 120 ml of rice milk
- 2 large pears
- 2 tablespoons of chopped hazelnuts to decorate

DIRECTIONS

1. Start by pouring all the dry ingredients into a large bowl: the flour, the organic lemon zest, the yeast and the salt and mix to make sure that everything comes together well.
2. Then add the liquids, then the rice milk and maple syrup and mix again until you get a soft and homogeneous consistency.
3. Meanwhile, peel and wash the two pears.
4. At this point, add the pears that you have previously cut into cubes, coarsely enough and mix to mix everything.

5. Now transfer the mixture into the cups inside a muffin mold and, before baking, sprinkle your muffins with little chopped hazelnuts.

6. Bake at 180 ° C for about 30 minutes in a static oven.

7. When they will be ready, let them cool and serve.

Coconut apple and walnut muffins

PREPARATION TIME: 15 minutes
COOKING TIME: 30 minutes
CALORIES: 415

INGREDIENTS FOR 4 SERVINGS

- 250 grams of wholemeal flour

- 50 grams of coconut flour

- zest of an untreated organic orange

- 120 ml of maple syrup

- 1 sachet of cream of tartar

- 1 pinch of salt

- 120 ml of sunflower oil

- 120 ml of coconut milk

- 2 large apples

- 2 tablespoons of chopped walnuts to decorate

DIRECTIONS

1. Start by pouring all the dry ingredients into a large bowl: the 2 flours, the organic orange zest, the yeast and the salt and mix to make sure that everything comes together well.

2. Then add the liquids, then the coconut milk and maple syrup and mix again until you get a soft and homogeneous consistency.

3. Meanwhile, peel and wash the two apples.

4. At this point, add the apples that you have previously cut into cubes, coarsely enough and mix to mix everything.

5. Now transfer the mixture into the cups inside a muffin mold and, before baking, sprinkle your muffins with little chopped hazelnuts.

6. Bake at 180 ° C for about 30 minutes in a static oven.

7. When they will be ready, let them cool and serve.

Apple and soy muffins

PREPARATION TIME: 15 minutes
COOKING TIME: 20 minutes
CALORIES: 335

INGREDIENTS FOR 4 SERVINGS

- 200 grams of wholemeal flour
- 200 grams of oat flour
- 1 large apple
- 250 grams of soy yogurt
- 240 ml of soymilk
- 100 grams of vegan whole cane sugar
- 120 ml of corn oil
- 1 sachet of natural yeast based on cream of tartar (16 grams)
- grated lemon zest
- juice of half a lemon

DIRECTIONS

1. Peel and cut the apple pulp into cubes.
2. Sprinkle apple cubes with lemon juice,
3. Now, dedicate yourself to the dough.
4. In a large bowl put the oat and wholemeal flour, the yeast and the sugar in which you have grated the lemon peel. In another bowl, add the yogurt, oil and soymilk: mix well until they are well blended.

5. Mix the powders with the liquids until you get a homogeneous mixture: now add the apple cubes.

6. Pour the mixture into cups placed in muffin molds, decorated with a few pieces of chopped almonds and bake everything at 180 °, static oven, for 20 minutes.

7. Remove from the oven, let cool and serve.

Apple and chocolate muffins

PREPARATION TIME: 15 minutes
COOKING TIME: 20 minutes
CALORIES: 390

INGREDIENTS FOR 4 SERVINGS

- 200 grams of wholemeal flour
- 100 grams of oat flour
- 100 grams of sugar free cocoa powder
- 1 large apple
- 250 grams of soy yogurt
- 240 ml of oat milk
- 100 grams of vegan whole cane sugar
- 20 grams of dark chocolate vegan chips
- 120 ml of vegetable oil
- 1 sachet of natural yeast based on cream of tartar (16 grams)
- grated lemon zest
- juice of half a lemon

DIRECTIONS

1. Peel and cut the apple pulp into cubes.
2. Sprinkle apple cubes with lemon juice,
3. Now, dedicate yourself to the dough.
4. In a large bowl put the oat and wholemeal flour, the cocoa powder, the yeast and the sugar in which you have grated the lemon peel.

5. In another bowl, add the yogurt, oil and oat milk: mix well until they are well blended.

6. Mix the powders with the liquids until you get a homogeneous mixture: now add the apple cubes and vegan chocolate chips.

7. Pour the mixture into cups placed in muffin molds, decorated with a few pieces of chopped almonds and bake everything at 180 °, static oven, for 20 minutes.

8. Remove from the oven, let cool and serve.

Apple and red fruits muffins

PREPARATION TIME: 15 minutes
COOKING TIME: 20 minutes
CALORIES: 360

INGREDIENTS FOR 4 SERVINGS

- 75 grams of oat flour
- 200 grams of wholemeal flour
- 100 grams of raw vegan cane sugar
- ½ sachet of yeast - (cream of tartar)
- ½ teaspoon of cinnamon
- 200 ml of almond milk
- 70 grams of sunflower oil
- ½ large apple
- 50 g of red fruits
- 1 pinch of salt

DIRECTIONS

1. In a bowl, mix the two types of flour, brown sugar, baking powder, cinnamon and salt.
2. Then add the almond milk and sunflower oil and mix just as necessary to obtain a homogeneous mixture.
3. Wash red fruits and let them dry.
4. Peel and cut the apple into small cubes and add it to the muffin mixture along with the red fruits and incorporate them, stirring a little more.
5. Now you can bake muffins

6. Cover your muffin molds with paper cups and fill them 3/4 of the way with the dough.

7. Then bake in a static oven at 190 ° C for 20 minutes about.

8. Once cooked, take them out of the oven and let them cool completely before enjoying them.

Peach and strawberry muffins

PREPARATION TIME: 15 minutes
COOKING TIME: 20 minutes
CALORIES: 380

INGREDIENTS FOR 4 SERVINGS

- 250 grams of wholemeal flour
- 25 grams of almond flour
- 100 grams of raw vegan cane sugar
- ½ sachet of yeast - (cream of tartar)
- ½ teaspoon of vanilla powder
- 200 ml of almond milk
- 70 grams of sunflower oil
- 1 small peach
- 70 grams of strawberries
- 1 pinch of salt

DIRECTIONS

1. In a bowl, mix the two types of flour, brown sugar, baking powder, vanilla powder and salt.
2. Then add the almond milk and sunflower oil and mix just as necessary to obtain a homogeneous mixture.
3. Wash strawberries and let them dry.
4. Peel and cut the peach into small cubes and add it to the muffin mixture along with the strawberries and incorporate them, stirring a little more.
5. Now you can bake muffins

6. Cover your muffin molds with paper cups and fill them 3/4 of the way with the dough.

7. Then bake in a static oven at 190 ° C for 20 minutes about.

8. Once cooked, take them out of the oven and let them cool completely before enjoying them.

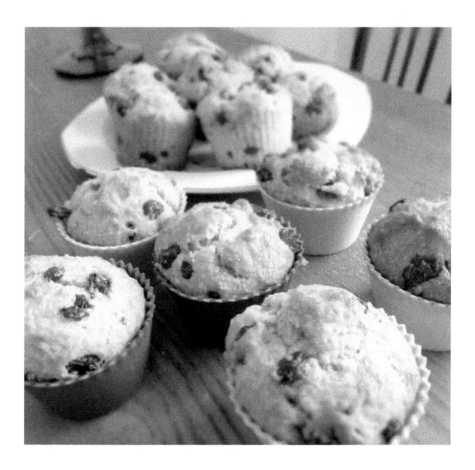

Orange and raisins muffins

PREPARATION TIME: 15 minutes
COOKING TIME: 30 minutes
CALORIES: 340

INGREDIENTS FOR 6/8 SERVINGS

- 300 grams of wholemeal flour
- 1 pinch of salt
- 1 sachet of cream of tartar
- 1 teaspoon of cinnamon
- 50 ml of orange juice
- 120 grams of maple or agave syrup
- 120 grams of corn oil
- 100 grams of raisins

DIRECTIONS

1. First, soak the raisins in warm water for at least 10 minutes.
2. At the same time, combine the dry ingredients of the recipe in a large bowl and mix together: then add the flour, the teaspoon of cinnamon, a pinch of salt and the cream of tartar.
3. In another bowl, add the liquid ingredients, then the oil, orange juice and maple syrup.
4. Then add the soaking raisins.
5. Take the liquids, add them to the powders and start mixing.
6. If the dough is too dry, you can add a drop of orange juice.

7. Take your mini muffin pan and, with the help of a spoon, pour the mixture directly into the pan or into the cups, if you use them.
8. You will need to bake the muffins for 30 minutes in a static oven at 180 ° C.
9. Let to cool, remove from the mold and serve.

Orange and hazelnut muffins

PREPARATION TIME: 15 minutes
COOKING TIME: 30 minutes
CALORIES: 380

INGREDIENTS FOR 6/8 SERVINGS

- 200 grams of wholemeal flour
- 100 grams of soy flour
- 1 pinch of salt
- 1 sachet of cream of tartar
- 1 teaspoon of nutmeg
- 50 ml of orange juice
- 80 grams of chopped hazelnuts
- 120 grams of maple syrup
- 120 grams of corn oil

DIRECTIONS

1. First, peel and chop very coarsely the hazelnuts.
2. At the same time, combine the dry ingredients of the recipe in a large bowl and mix: then add the wholemeal flour, the soy flour, nutmeg, a pinch of salt and the cream of tartar.
3. In another bowl, add the liquid ingredients, then the oil, orange juice and maple syrup.
4. Then add the chopped hazelnuts.
5. Take the liquids, add them to the powders and start mixing.

6. If the dough is too dry, you can add a drop of orange juice.

7. Take your mini muffin pan and, with the help of a spoon, pour the mixture directly into the pan or into the cups, if you use them.

8. You will need to bake the muffins for 30 minutes in a static oven at 180 ° C.

9. Let to cool, remove from the mold and serve.

Coconut and chocolate muffins

PREPARATION TIME: 15 minutes
COOKING TIME: 30 minutes
CALORIES: 480

INGREDIENTS FOR 4 SERVINGS

- 200 grams of wholemeal flour
- 150 grams of coconut flour
- 1 pinch of salt
- 1 sachet of natural yeast based on cream of tartar (16 g)
- 150 ml of maple syrup
- 120 ml of sunflower oil
- 160 ml of coconut milk
- 20 grams of chopped almonds
- 100 grams of vegan dark chocolate

DIRECTIONS

1. Start the recipe by preparing the dough
2. Sift all the dry ingredients into a large bowl: the 2 flours and the yeast, then add the salt and mix.
3. In another bowl, prepare the liquids: maple syrup, sunflower oil and coconut milk.
4. Add the liquid ingredients to the dry ones and mix well until you get a soft and homogeneous dough without lumps.

5. Separately, put the dark chocolate in a bowl and melt it in a double boiler in a saucepan with water over medium heat.

6. Once the chocolate has melted, add it to your dough and mix to mix everything well.

7. Meanwhile peel and chop very finely almonds.

8. Pour the mixture into muffin molds and, before baking, sprinkle the muffins with chopped almonds over.

9. At this point, cook in a static oven at 180ºC for about 25/30 minutes.

10. Let double chocolate muffins cool and serve.

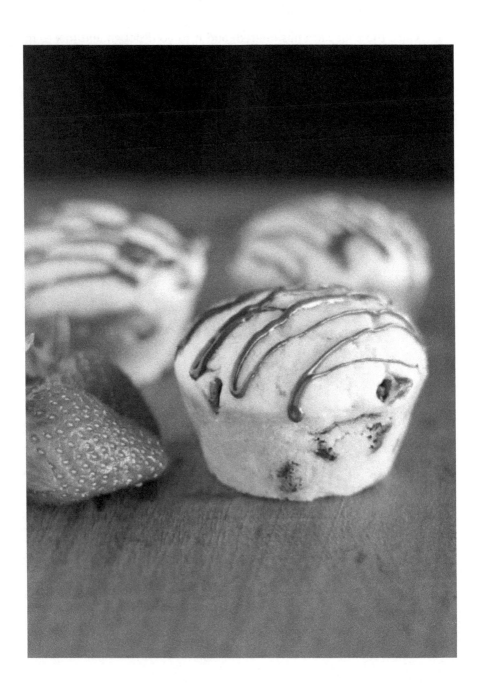

Lightning Source UK Ltd.
Milton Keynes UK
UKHW010654240621
386081UK00010B/503